Teamwork, Leadership and Communication

Teamwork, Leadership and Communication

Collaboration Basics for
Health Professionals

DEBORAH LAKE, PHD
KRISTA BAERG, BSN, MD
TERESA PASLAWSKI, PHD

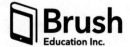

Editorial: Ruth Bradley-St-Cyr, Shauna Babiuk
Cover: Dean Pickup; Cover Image: © Yang Yu | Dreamstime.com
Interior Design: Carol Dragich, Dragich Design

Brush Education Inc.
www.brusheducation.ca
contact@brusheducation.ca

Printed and manufactured in Canada

Library and Archives Canada Cataloguing in Publication

Lake, Deborah, 1950-, author

    Teamwork, leadership and communication : collaboration basics for health professionals / Deborah Lake, PhD, Krista Baerg, MD, Teresa Paslawski, PhD.

Includes bibliographical references and index.
Issued in print and electronic formats.
ISBN 978-1-55059-640-3 (paperback).—ISBN 978-1-55059-641-0 (pdf).—
ISBN 978-1-55059-642-7 (mobi).—ISBN 978-1-55059-643-4 (epub)

    1. Health care teams. 2. Interprofessional relations. 3. Communication in medicine. 4. Leadership. 5. Medical personnel. I. Baerg, Krista, 1969-, author II. Paslawski, Teresa, 1967-, author III. Title.

R729.5.H4L34 2015   610.69   C2015-902650-4
                                            C2015-902651-2

We acknowledge the support of the Government of Canada.
Nous reconnaissons l'appui du gouvernement du Canada.

Contents

Acknowledgments

This book grew out of several early projects on interprofessional collaboration, including leading hands-on workshops for students and/or practicing professionals, publishing the results of an online survey, and developing teaching modules. We thank those who participated in these projects for their engagement, stories, and insights. We also thank our students, research associates, and colleagues for their contributions, in particular Cara Zukewich. We are grateful for the institutional and financial support we have received for our early work, including funding by Health Canada through Patient-Centered Interprofessional Team Experiences (P-CITE) at the University of Saskatchewan. We acknowledge the support of the three universities with which the authors are currently affiliated: the University of Manitoba, the University of Saskatchewan, and the University of Alberta.

Melva McLean, editor, provided valuable guidance after reviewing an early draft of this book. Many other readers offered suggestions for our vignettes. The Brush Education publishing team has been accommodating, creative, and resourceful. We are indebted to our family members who sustained us throughout this work.

We take responsibility for any errors or misinterpretations contained in this book and welcome suggestions and comments from readers. The vignettes we constructed are fabrications or distillations of our collective experience — any resemblance to real individuals or situations is coincidental.

Preface

There has been a surge of attention, even a paradigm shift, toward interprofessional collaboration (IPC) in healthcare over the past few decades. Collaboration has been identified as a core role for health professionals and IPC competencies have been delineated. Professional regulatory bodies have added IPC principles to their standards of professional practice. Accrediting bodies include IPC benchmarks in their requirements for healthcare services and professional education programs. Hospitals and other healthcare organizations provide training and administrative support to improve IPC. New journals focus on IPC research, theory, and practice. As well, health professionals increasingly provide services in non-traditional settings, such as schools, requiring collaboration with professionals from other fields.

Despite this paradigm shift, opportunities for health professionals and students to develop fundamental competencies in IPC may be haphazard. Whether IPC is introduced in interprofessional education experiences or in discipline-specific courses on professional issues, attention to basic attitudes, values, skills, and knowledge varies widely across institutions and professions. In addition, students may be evaluated on their IPC competencies by clinical supervisors with limited knowledge of this area. For practicing health professionals, continuing education or in-service training for IPC must compete with many other important topics for scarce professional development time and resources.

Convincing health professionals and students to devote time to developing IPC skills may be difficult since most people believe they already know how to collaborate. Even so, the attitudes, skills, and knowledge that contribute to successful collaboration are not innate or instinctive, as anyone watching a group of squabbling preschool children can attest. Over time, we learn how to work cooperatively with others and most of us learn these skills implicitly through experience. Because each person has a unique history of collaboration experiences, each person brings different expectations to IPC in healthcare. These different expectations can lead to confusion, frustration, conflict, and low productivity. Precisely because of these different expectations, health professionals engaged in IPC require retraining so that they may build shared mental models of their work together — shared mental models that lead to success.

The three authors of this book came from different professions to form a working group for a series of projects related to IPC in healthcare. What united us further was a firm belief that skillful IPC requires explicit training rather than mere exposure. Exposing students to interprofessional education experiences without guiding their acquisition of core IPC competencies is analogous to putting desks in a classroom and assuming that people will learn simply by sitting at the desks. When learners develop IPC competencies within a supportive environment and a systematic framework, they become adept at handling the situations they will encounter throughout their professional lives (Roegiers, 2007).

We offer this book as a resource to those who wish to improve their practice of IPC. To promote a shared understanding of IPC, we have focused on core competencies that transcend professional roles and national boundaries. This book will be useful to healthcare students, practicing health professionals, professionals from other fields who collaborate with health professionals, and healthcare administrators who support collaborative care environments. To promote active learning, each chapter has a variety of exercises, suggestions for reflection, links to online resources, and vignettes of common experiences in healthcare.

In this book, we organize IPC competencies into three broad domains: teamwork, leadership, and communication (TLC). These three domains emerged from our review of the extensive literature on IPC as well as our own research (Baerg, Lake, & Paslawski, 2012). The initials *TLC* bring to mind their traditional use as a short form for *tender loving care*, which is as important in collaboration as it is in patient care. As well, we invite readers to consider each of these competency domains at three levels of context: interpersonal, organizational, and systemic. This framework for conceptualizing three domains of IPC competencies at three levels can be used as a tool for learning, reflection, and problem solving.

Scattered throughout the book are storm cloud graphics containing comments that express some negative perceptions of IPC. These comments were collected from pre-service healthcare students who had participated in introductory IPC courses (Paslawski, 2013). We include these comments in recognition of the confusion, resistance, or frustration that IPC may generate from time to time. We hope that you find within these pages the insights and practical tools to lead you through those clouds to experiences of clarity, encouragement, and success.

I like IPC but I don't want any training.

To meet the challenge of writing for a diverse audience, we have chosen familiar terms commonly used across most health professions.

For example, we use the term *patient* for the recipient of healthcare, recognizing that patients are not just recipients of care but also collaborate with health professionals. We sometimes use other terms such as *client* in specific examples or vignettes to preserve their authenticity. We use the term *interprofessional* in the broadest sense of collaboration across professions, reserving the term *interdisciplinary* for a specific type of team structure. Finally, we have drawn on sources from the fields of education, organizational development, and business. These fields have their own terminology, which we have sometimes adapted to fit the purpose of this book.

Dave Barry, the popular humorist, said, "The one thing that unites all human beings, regardless of age, gender, religion, economic status or ethnic background, is that, deep down inside, we ALL believe that we are above average drivers" (Barry, 1998, p. 182). In our own research (Baerg et al., 2012), most participants rated themselves as having above average skills in teamwork, leadership, and communication, but they also stated they had little knowledge of these areas as they relate to IPC. The purpose of this book is to provide this knowledge so readers may indeed develop above average skills.

Introduction

Imagine working with a group of people who trust each other and share common goals. They know they can weather episodes of confusion or conflict — in fact, they understand that such episodes can lead to new understandings and result in decisions that everyone can support...

AFTER READING THIS CHAPTER, YOU WILL BE ABLE TO DO THE FOLLOWING:

- Define *interprofessional collaboration in healthcare* and distinguish collaboration from consultation
- Justify the central role of *patient- and family-centered care* in interprofessional collaboration
- Explain the *rationale* for collaborating in healthcare
- Map out a *framework* for understanding collaboration competencies and challenges in various contexts

Interprofessional collaboration has become a cornerstone of modern healthcare. Since collaboration is a social process, its course is not always smooth. To be efficacious, interprofessional collaboration requires participants who are willing, knowledgeable, and skilled, as well as settings that provide opportunities and resources. While settings vary, participants can transfer their attitudes, skills, and knowledge from one setting to another. Moreover, knowledgeable participants understand how the setting affects their collaboration and have the skills to adapt to different settings, especially when working collaboratively with patients and their families. Finally, mature health professionals understand that their competencies for interprofessional collaboration are continuously evolving.

Interprofessional Collaboration in Healthcare

Various models, definitions, and descriptions of interprofessional collaboration in healthcare (Canadian Interprofessional Health Collaborative, 2009;

D'Amour & Oandasan, 2005; Way, Jones, & Busing, 2000; World Health Organization, 2010) point to the following essential components:

- A process for communicating and making decisions
- Shared goals
- The whole is more than the sum of its parts (synergy)

More specifically, "to collaborate is to create conversations in which people are joined together, meanings are fashioned, purposes are defined, roles are clarified, goals are established, and action is taken" (Seaburn, Lorenz, Gunn, Gawinski, & Mauksch, 1996, p. 9).

EXERCISE 1.1

Review the following online resources to find models and definitions for interprofessional collaboration and interprofessional education:

American Interprofessional Health Collaborative: www.aihc-us.org/

Canadian Interprofessional Health Collaborative: www.cihc.ca/

Centre for the Advancement of Interprofessional Education (UK): www.caipe.org.uk/

Framework for action on interprofessional education and collaborative practice (World Health Organization, 2010): www.who.int/hrh/resources /framework_action/en/

What are some common threads among these organizations?

_____

_____

_____

What resources may be especially useful for you and your setting?

_____

_____

_____

In healthcare, collaboration and consultation are commonly used terms that are not interchangeable. Consultation is a process of seeking information from others in which the seeker integrates new information and generates a plan while retaining control of the process. In practice, the process of consultation becomes increasingly complicated as medical complexity increases and more professionals are involved. As a result, the patient may receive conflicting information or advice from different professionals. Collaboration, on the other hand, is characterized by joint goal setting and shared decision making and, when patient and family centered, with the patient and family as active participants. Effective collaboration results in shared understandings and plans supported by all participants.

Interprofessional collaboration is ideal but incredibly difficult!

Goals of collaboration in healthcare usually relate in some way to patient care, health, and well-being. Providing collaborative care to patients may be direct or indirect, as the following examples illustrate:

- Joint goal setting and care plan development for a hospitalized patient during bedside rounds
- A discharge-planning meeting with a hospital patient, community-based services, and family members
- A meeting to revise outdated patient-education handouts
- An ad hoc committee to organize in-service professional training
- A meeting between health professionals and school-based support services regarding a child with complex medical and social needs
- A research group working on a quality-improvement project
- A meeting with administration to respond to organizational policy changes that affect patient care

Professionals might be involved in several of these activities within the span of a few days. As Ho wrote in the *Journal of Interprofessional Care*, collaboration "is fundamental to the very fabric of the careers of health professionals" (2008, p. 1).

As health professionals, we may work with others from our own profession (intraprofessional collaboration) or from different professions (interprofessional collaboration). Working with individuals from other professions allows us to capitalize on the different perspectives each profession brings to the task. Just as we can see a visual illusion differently with the help of another person (see Figure 1.1), we can see a patient, problem, or task differently with the help of someone from a different profession. As the complexity of a patient, problem, or task increases, so does the need to incorporate multiple perspectives to ensure that this complexity is addressed.

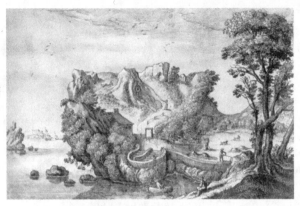

FIGURE 1.1 VISUAL ILLUSION

EXERCISE 1.2

Identify some other examples of situations or kinds of work that require health professionals to collaborate.

Is there a clear distinction between collaboration and consultation in these examples?

_____

_____

_____

If not, how would you clarify expectations for your work?

_____

_____

_____

Patient- and Family-Centered Care

Patient- and family-centered care is central to emerging models of collaboration in healthcare (Canadian Interprofessional Health Collaborative, 2009; D'Amour & Oandasan, 2005; Leathard, 2003). While patient- and family-centered care is widely endorsed, it is not easily defined. As Stewart has noted, patient-centered care "may be most commonly understood for what it is not — technology centred, doctor centred, hospital centred, disease centred"

(2001, p. 444). In patient- and family-centered care, patient and family priorities drive care delivery following a biopsychosocial model (Borrell-Carrio, Suchman, & Epstein, 2004). Because people outside the healthcare system often have different points of view from those of insiders, patient- and family-centered care obliges professionals to be open to seeing things from new perspectives.

The core concepts of patient- and family-centered care are respect and dignity, information sharing, participation, and collaboration (Institute for Patient- and Family-Centered Care, 2010a). These same concepts are fundamental to interprofessional collaboration. Professionals who work at improving their skills for interprofessional collaboration will also enhance their skills for patient- and family-centered care: they will more successfully engage patients in collaborative decision making so that the promise of "nothing about me without me" is fulfilled (Wynia, Von Kohorn, & Mitchell, 2012, p. 1327).

EXERCISE 1.3

Explore the website for the Institute for Patient- and Family-Centered Care, especially responses to common questions about patient- and family-centered care on their FAQ page,[1] and then answer the following questions:

What is meant by the word family?

_____

_____

_____

Does patient- and family-centered care take more time?

_____

_____

_____

Does patient- and family-centered care cost more?

_____

_____

_____

The extent to which collaborative healthcare is patient- and family-centered can be measured by the decisions and outcomes (e.g., treatment plans) of the group. Groups with members predisposed to considering different perspectives are more likely to come up with more comprehensive patient- and family-centered treatment plans. However, it is not sufficient merely to have different professional perspectives represented; the decision-making process of the group must allow each person's perspective to influence the outcome. A favorable and satisfying outcome of effective collaborative practice is its synergistic effect. As one healthcare provider commented, "Putting our minds together and coming up with new ideas is enriching" (Way, Jones, & Busing, 2000, p. 4). When each person's perspectives influence the outcome, all group members have more confidence in the result.

Interprofessional collaboration implies that I don't have enough knowledge or experience to do the work myself.

Rationale

J. Richard Hackman, editor of the 1990 book *Groups that Work (and Those that Don't),* points out the following:

> Some tasks . . . cannot be done if there is not a group to perform them. Examples include performing a string quartet, safely flying a Boeing 727, and playing a baseball game. Other tasks, however, are almost always accomplished by an individual rather than by a group. No great poem has ever been written by a team; few paradigm-shattering scientific theories are group products; and there are not many group-composed symphonic scores. (p. xiii)

It is easy to think of healthcare tasks and activities that can and should be done independently. It is more difficult for health professionals to agree when collaboration is needed and to have the flexibility to respond collaboratively in complex organizational and interpersonal environments, especially when changing patient needs require a quick response. A well-accepted principle is that interprofessional collaboration "is essential when patient needs and problems are multiple, complex and/or overlap professional boundaries" (Heinemann, Schmitt, Farrell, & Brallier, 1999, p. 123). One of the reasons interprofessional collaboration is difficult to do well is that the kinds of problems that require collaboration are often intrinsically difficult.

Understandably, assessing the efficacy of collaboration in healthcare is a complex undertaking. Nevertheless, important progress has been made, as the following examples illustrate:

- Effective collaborative care has been found to lead to reduced readmission rates to hospitals (Sommers, Marton, Barbaccia, & Randolph, 2000), lower costs (Curley, McEachern, & Speroff, 1998), and improved patient care (Zwarenstein, Goldman, & Reeves, 2009).
- Meta-analyses of geriatric team interventions have found a significantly reduced mortality risk, an increased likelihood of living at home, and improved physical and cognitive function at various intervals post-hospitalization (Schmitt, 2001).
- Team effectiveness was associated with successful implementation of an innovative strategy to enhance access to clinical care in US Veterans Affairs medical centers (Lukas, Mohr, & Meterko, 2009).
- Teamwork training has been shown to improve patient safety by reducing adverse outcomes and errors in emergency departments, operating rooms, obstetrics units, and outpatient primary care clinics (Agency for Healthcare Research and Quality, 2014).

The benefits of improving interprofessional collaboration can be substantial. This body of research also indicates that the quality of interprofessional collaboration is important: launching a collaborative approach with no regard for how people work together does not guarantee success. Moreover, much of the research demonstrating the benefits of interprofessional collaboration in healthcare is based on one-time projects or initiatives. The extent to which sustained benefits accrue from pre-licensure education and post-licensure interventions is less clear (Zwarenstein, Reeves, & Perrier, 2005).

I don't think much gets accomplished.

Research on the outcomes of patient- and family-centered care has a similar pattern to the research described above on outcomes of interprofessional collaboration initiatives. Although the efficacy of interventions to promote patient-centered care is well established (Stacey et al., 2014), information on the sustainability and effectiveness of coordinated patient-centered care in real clinical practice is still emerging (Barry & Edgman-Levitan, 2012; Wagner & Groves, 2002). Like interprofessional collaboration, providing patient-centered care is an interpersonal process with barriers and enablers at organizational and systemic levels (Suter, Deutschlander, & Lait, 2011).

EXERCISE 1.4

Develop a 15-second elevator speech to convince a colleague that inter-professional collaboration is essential to effective healthcare.

What barriers or misconceptions must you address?

_____

_____

_____

When systems for accreditation and regulation establish standards for interprofessional collaboration, they promote its sustainability and strengthen the health system overall (World Health Organization, 2010). There are many examples of how such systems are carrying this mission forward. Accrediting bodies for hospitals and community health services now incorporate standards for interprofessional collaboration into their policies and requirements (Accreditation Canada, 2014; Joint Commission, 2013). Many healthcare professional associations include principles or standards for interprofessional collaboration among their core competencies for professional practice (American Nurses Association/American Organization of Nurse Executives, n.d.; General Dental Council, 2011; Royal College of Physicians and Surgeons of Canada, 2005). More broadly, representatives of various health professions have come together to generate competency frameworks for interprofessional collaboration (Canadian Interprofessional Health Collaborative, 2010; Interprofessional Education Collaborative Expert Panel, 2011; Interprofessional Education Team, 2010). In turn, these competency frameworks are being translated into accreditation standards for healthcare education programs (AIPHE, 2011; see also Zorek & Raehl, 2013). The emergence of these standards and frameworks reflects our growing understanding of the importance of interprofessional collaboration to enhance performance, prevent errors, and improve clinical outcomes in healthcare. These systemic changes are part of a necessary and timely redesign of professional health education (Frenk et al., 2010).

Framework

In this book, we have employed a back-to-basics approach by identifying and focusing on three competency domains that are fundamental to effective collaboration: teamwork, leadership, and communication (TLC). In our framework, teamwork competencies include attitudes toward working with others, interpersonal skills, and knowledge of group dynamics. Leadership competencies include knowledge of shared leadership and participatory decision making, leadership skills, and conflict management. Communication competencies include understanding how communication in groups differs from dyadic communication, self-awareness, and communication skills (e.g., active listening).

For any given collaborative enterprise, there are three levels of context: interpersonal, organizational, and systemic. The interpersonal level is specific to a group of individuals: their roles, characteristics, needs, and goals. The organizational level is specific to the immediate working context: a hospital, practice, clinic, business, or regional health authority. The systemic level encompasses a much larger context: professional and legal standards, geographic location, population changes, culture, and time frame.

The intersection of three competency domains with three levels of context results in a simple matrix (see Table 1.1). This matrix provides a framework for thinking about collaboration and for improving collaboration capacity. It is useful for both beginners and experienced professionals, for individuals and groups. The matrix can be used as a pedagogical tool to structure learning or as a problem-solving tool to pinpoint breakdowns in the collaborative process. In the end, the matrix is useful as an easy-to-remember framework: three competency domains (teamwork, leadership, and communication) at three levels of operation (interpersonal, organizational, and systemic).

TABLE 1.1 FRAMEWORK OF COMPETENCY DOMAINS AND LEVELS OF OPERATION

	INTERPERSONAL	ORGANIZATIONAL	SYSTEMIC
Teamwork			
Leadership			
Communication			

Each of the next three chapters provides three vignettes of common experiences in healthcare. These nine vignettes illustrate issues in teamwork, leadership, and communication in different contexts. While each vignette highlights one cell of the framework, perceptive readers will notice that other competencies and levels of context may be relevant. As you work through each vignette, we invite you to think outside the box and apply this framework as you see fit.

EXERCISE 1.5

Appreciative inquiry: Briefly describe one positive experience you have had with collaboration. You may draw from any context — professional, volunteer, educational, recreational, and so on.

What made this experience positive for you?

_____

_____

_____

Select two elements of this positive experience and consider where they might fit in the framework — which row or which column?

_____

_____

_____

NOTE

1 www.ipfcc.org/faq.html

2

Teamwork

Imagine a meeting filled with energy, optimism, humor, and respect. People attending this meeting value the time they spend together and use that time well . . .

AFTER READING THIS CHAPTER, YOU WILL BE ABLE TO DO THE FOLLOWING:

- Understand the importance of *positive attitudes* toward working with others
- Address concerns about *liability*
- Recognize core *interpersonal skills* for teamwork
- Explain how *group dynamics* affect group performance, including the size, composition, structure, context, and development of the group
- *Apply the framework* to understand challenges in teamwork

Teamwork is the combined action of a group of people. The paradox of teamwork is that it relies on the individual skills of those sharing responsibility (Avery, 2001). To be good at teamwork, you need positive attitudes toward working with others and a range of interpersonal skills. You also need to understand how group dynamics are affected by the group's size, composition, context, structure (e.g., multidisciplinary, interdisciplinary, or transdisciplinary), and changes over time. Skilled collaborators continually and intentionally work on their teamwork attitudes, skills, and knowledge, which don't develop without effort.

Attitudes toward Working with Others

Collaborative work is driven by the energy and enthusiasm of its participants. But even the most enthusiastic champions of collaboration acknowledge that it is hard work and not always completely satisfying. For action-oriented people, the process of working with others may feel slow and needlessly complicated: time spent developing collaborative relationships may feel like a diversion from "real" work. Even those who thrive on working with others may become discouraged when the group gets stuck, distracted, divisive, or unfocused.

To sustain effort through difficult times, it is important for everyone involved to be convinced of the importance of collaboration in relation to his or her own goals and needs. Some people may be persuaded of this importance by reading the extensive research literature that justifies collaboration in business, healthcare, education, and other human service sectors. Others may prefer to think through the particulars of the task to understand why collaboration is the best approach: why they need the input of others with different roles, knowledge, ideas, experiences, and/or training. Still others may reflect on previous energizing, effective, and empowering experiences with collaboration. In any case, it doesn't hurt to have at least one cheerleader in the group: a champion of collaboration who reminds the others of their reasons for working together. Enthusiasm for the group and its potential to achieve its goals can be contagious.

I have a solo working style, so I don't like interprofessional collaboration.

A valuable tool for assessing attitudes to teamwork in healthcare is the Attitudes toward Health Care Teams Scale (Heinemann et al., 1999). Research using this scale with practicing professionals and trainees has found positive attitudes across professions toward the value and efficiency of healthcare teams (Heinemann et al., 1999; Hyer, Fairchild, Abraham, Mezey, & Fulmer, 2000; Leipzig et al., 2002). This same research revealed disagreement about the role of physicians in healthcare teams. For example, compared with practitioners from other health professions, physicians and physician trainees agreed more with statements like this one: "The physician has the right to alter patient care plans developed by the team." When group members honestly identify and openly discuss their expectations and convictions about professional roles and responsibilities, they anticipate potential conflicts. In many situations, medical practitioners must balance their role as a collaborator with their role as the most responsible physician (Whitehead, 2007); frank discussion of these roles increases group members' awareness of this balance.

Liability

Physicians and other professionals may fear that sharing responsibility puts them at increased risk for liability. Indeed, liability can arise from negligent acts due to lack of clarity regarding roles and responsibilities that "lead to *inappropriate delegation of duties* or *abdication of responsibility* [emphasis in original]" (Conference Board of Canada, 2007, p. ii). A review of relevant court cases in the United States and Canada by the Conference Board of

EXERCISE 2.1

Complete the Attitudes toward Health Care Teams Scale reprinted in
Appendix A. Compare your results with those of someone from another
profession OR complete the scale again from the point of view of a person
from a different profession.

What similarities do you have? Where do you disagree?

_____

_____

_____

*What can you learn from the other person about their reasons for
responding differently from you?*

_____

_____

_____

*Regardless of your profession, what situation might lead you to change a
patient care plan developed by the team?*

_____

_____

_____

Canada revealed that liability is not a barrier to interprofessional collaboration when all professionals follow these guidelines:

- Act according to their professional standards and comply with regula-
  tions set by their regulatory bodies
- Work within teams to clarify roles and responsibilities, and set policies
  and procedures for communication, decision making, and patient management

- Understand their scope of practice and limitations as set out in relevant legislation
- Understand the scopes of practice of other professionals on their team
- Understand and comply with policies that govern their interdisciplinary interactions, especially when there is role overlap
- Maintain appropriate malpractice liability insurance
- Ensure that the organization has malpractice liability insurance that covers the organization and its employees (e.g., direct liability, vicarious liability)

Overall, major healthcare stakeholders agree that the potential of collaborative care models to enhance the delivery of healthcare should not be hindered by unfounded fears of increased liability (Canadian Medical Protective Association, 2008).

Attitudes shape our behavior. To collaborate effectively, you need to be aware of your own attitudes toward teamwork as well as those of your colleagues. Fortunately, attitudes toward teamwork are not etched in stone — they change with new experiences and insights. When team members have conversations about their attitudes toward teamwork, they build a shared understanding about their work together. Those conversations are more likely to be positive if all participants employ key interpersonal skills.

Interpersonal Skills

Good working relationships are built on trust. To collaborate, people need to trust one another enough to share their vulnerabilities as well as their strengths — what they don't know as well as what they do know, what they can't do as well as what they can do. Collaborators build trust over time using a range of interpersonal skills. Specifically, they show respect, establish rapport, demonstrate commitment, and cooperate.

I didn't like the people I was working with.

When co-workers show respect, they affirm the value of each person in the working relationship. It is not necessary for all group members to like each other (Avery, 2001, p. 21). Rather, group members recognize that shared responsibility requires attention to the quality of respect in relationships. For interprofessional groups, this quality of respect includes recognizing the importance of the expertise contributed by each profession or discipline. For patient- and family-centered care, this quality of respect includes recognizing the values, beliefs, knowledge, and cultural context of patients and families — listening to their perspectives and honoring their choices.

Co-workers establish rapport by listening, showing warmth and empathy, being tactful and approachable, and having a sense of humor. Health professional education programs often provide specific training for building rapport with patients. Using these same skills to build rapport with co-workers is a sign of professional integrity. Those who build rapport with their co-workers also reap the benefits of increased trust and efficiency in collaboration.

Showing up, pitching in, and following through show commitment. Such commitment communicates respect for the goals and the other members of the group. Being mindful of the importance of honoring commitments helps one think twice about saying "yes" simply to be agreeable. Productivity and fulfillment thrive when group members can rely on each other to honor their commitments.

Finally, collaborators cooperate with others by being flexible and adaptable, although not at the expense of deeply held values or beliefs. Indeed, an important role of each member of a group is to prevent misguided groupthink by disagreeing in an honest and respectful manner. Cooperation includes being open to different points of view, compromising, and overlooking minor differences in style. Cooperation also includes responding to requests for assistance and offering to help.

When all members of a working group demonstrate respect, establish and maintain rapport, and show commitment and cooperation, a climate of mutual trust can develop quickly. Similarly, failure to build trust can inhibit or derail the work of the group. For some groups, time spent on trust-building exercises may be a good investment. One common trust-building exercise is to establish ground rules or trust efficiencies — a set of agreements to speed up the development of working relationships in the group (Avery, 2001, pp. 158–159). Such agreements clarify norms of the group for any or all of the following areas: attendance, preparation, participation, decision making, and follow-through.

Group Dynamics

Group dynamics are the interaction patterns specific to a group. While the personalities and attitudes of group members certainly contribute to group dynamics, the characteristics of the group as a whole are equally important. Group dynamics

VIGNETTE 2.1

A skilled therapist establishes rapport with a new client while his student and members of his interdisciplinary team observe from behind a one-way window. The therapist is warm and gentle, listens to the client, and paraphrases the client's concerns well. After leaving the clinic room, the therapist stuns other members of his team when he yells at his student, using coarse and belittling language.

What does the therapist's behavior reveal about his skills and attitudes?

How might the other members of the team feel about working with this therapist?

depend on the size of the group, its composition, its structure, its context and its development over time. Knowledge about these contributors to group dynamics provides a framework for understanding what is happening in a group.

Group Size

Research shows that group dynamics of small working groups differ from those of large working groups (Yeatts & Hyten, 1998, pp. 257–260). Small groups — about four to seven members — tend to have high cohesion and motivation leading to effective work performance. Members get to know each other well and each member tends to contribute to decision making, which enhances commitment both to each other and to the group's outcomes. On the other hand, small groups have fewer resources, leading to heavy workloads or possibly forcing members to assume roles beyond their capabilities or scope of practice.

> There is always at least one person on the team who does not do his or her share of the work.

Large groups have more resources but run the risk of reduced individual accountability or social loafing. Even if everyone is committed to the work, large groups require more time for communication and decision making. Large groups also run the risk of developing friction between subgroups or factions. Nevertheless, size alone does not doom a group to failure. Yeatts and Hyten (1998) described a case study of a high-performing 17-member group. They credited its success to several adaptations, including delegation of tasks to subgroups, an administrative structure that allowed for skilled coordination of subgroups, and maintenance of respect and status among group members through the larger organization's reward system.

What is the best size for a working group? The short answer is that the group should include all the stakeholders needed to accomplish the goal (Mattessich, Murray-Close, & Monsey, 2001, p. 16). Straus (2002, pp. 40–51) identified four types of stakeholders:

- Those with the formal power to make a decision
- Those with the power to block a decision
- Those affected by a decision
- Those with relevant information or expertise

Patients and family members are stakeholders in direct-care settings. At organizational and systemic levels, patient representatives provide a voice for those affected by decisions and thereby support patient- and family-centered care.

For larger projects with many stakeholders, individuals may participate at different "rings of involvement" (Straus, 2002, p. 48). Members of the core problem-solving group usually commit the greatest amount of time and energy. Others may participate in various activities, such as task forces, subcommittees, hearings, feedback or feed-forward meetings, and brainstorming sessions. For those least involved, communication can be through newsletters, email, and mass media. Straus noted the following:

> Often, if you extend an invitation to someone with an explanation of the time commitments required, the individual will feel acknowledged but opt for a less-intense ring of involvement. If you exclude that person, however, he or she may come pounding at the door. (2002, p. 50)

Such invitations to different rings of involvement can actually increase the participation of all stakeholders because they can see how to contribute without becoming overwhelmed.

Group Composition

Group composition refers to the characteristics of the people in the group. Collaboration typically thrives on diversity. Diversity may be achieved through role-related characteristics and/or personal characteristics of the group members. Role-related characteristics include occupation, organizational position, and specialized knowledge or skills. Personal characteristics include age, gender, family situation, nationality, cultural values, and personality.

Diversity of group membership can be a double-edged sword — it can both enhance and hinder group functioning. Research has shown that diversity of occupation and diversity of some personal characteristics are generally associated with positive effects, especially for tasks where considering different points of view is important. In contrast, diversity of rank, status, culture, or nationality has sometimes been associated with negative effects (Yeatts & Hyten, 1998, p. 263).

Equipped with this knowledge, group members may wish to address rank or status issues directly to improve group function and satisfaction. Team-building exercises can help counteract stereotyping among group members with different cultural backgrounds or nationalities. Targeted communication training may be of value for groups with diverse backgrounds. Social time together, such as sharing a meal, can help group members learn more about each other outside of the work context. This important topic is revisited in the chapters on leadership and communication.

Group Structure

The structure of the group refers to how its members interact to work toward their goal: communicating, planning, making decisions, maintaining records, and solving problems. The structure of short-term working groups is typically predetermined by the leadership; for example, a workshop leader or an organizer of a case conference. The structure of stable, long-term working groups may be predetermined or may emerge over time. Awareness of the group's structure is essential to collaboration and should be part of the orientation of each new member.

In healthcare, working groups are often organized as teams. Mosser and Begun (2014) distinguish between management teams and clinical teams, as well as different kinds of clinical teams. Management teams may have clinicians as members, but their work is to manage the delivery of healthcare services and supportive activities. Clinical teams interact directly with patients and families to provide patient care. According to Mosser and Begun (chap. 2), clinical teams can be further subdivided into the following subtypes:

- True teams have shared operational responsibility, clear leaders, and stable membership over time; for example, a chronic pain clinic team consisting of an anesthesiologist, a nurse, a physiotherapist, and a psychologist.
- Template teams have shared responsibility and clear leaders, but their membership changes over time, such as a surgical team drawn from a larger group of physicians, nurses, assistants, and technologists who step into highly specific and well-defined roles.
- Knotworks are groups with shared responsibility but no clear leader or stable membership, such as a one-time cluster of clinicians caring for a patient with complex and chronic problems.

While knotworks are common in healthcare, they are not considered teams because their membership is not clearly defined.

Teams that have people from different occupations or disciplines are typically grouped into one of three common structures: multidisciplinary, interdisciplinary, or transdisciplinary (see Figures 2.1, 2.2, and 2.3 for examples of each structure). The following descriptions are drawn from the work of Foley (1990).

Multidisciplinary teams are the most common and most varied. A multidisciplinary team may be set up intentionally with a clear structure or it may arise spontaneously with few set parameters. Typically, there is one person in charge, a gatekeeper who coordinates the team's activities and makes decisions. Communication flows through the coordinator and there may be little or no interaction between some of the team members. While some work may be done jointly, the predominant operating principle is one of parallel action.

On interdisciplinary teams, all members make important decisions and plans collaboratively. The function of the coordinator of an interdisciplinary team is to facilitate the work of the team rather than to make decisions. Communication flows freely among all team members, often in face-to-face meetings. While some activities may take place independently, the predominant operating principle is one of cooperation.

EXERCISE 2.2

Identify examples of true teams, template teams, and knotworks from your own experience.

Did each of these groups engage all stakeholders appropriately?

_____

_____

_____

What made the group work well?

_____

_____

_____

What challenges did it encounter?

_____

_____

_____

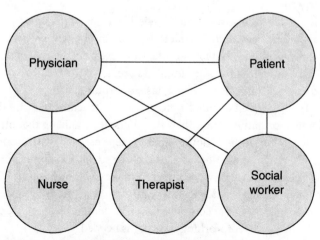

FIGURE 2.1 MULTIDISCIPLINARY TEAM STRUCTURE

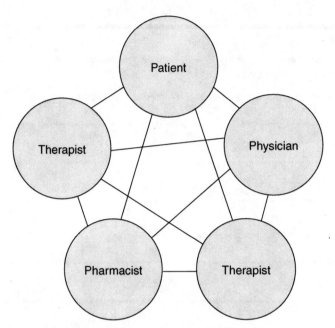

FIGURE 2.2 INTERDISCIPLINARY TEAM STRUCTURE

On transdisciplinary teams, individuals share expertise as they collaborate. Typically, transdisciplinary teams are formally organized with clear expectations of working in a way that transcends the usual discipline boundaries. Team members trust each other to carry out aspects of their own roles (known as role release) and spend time clarifying role boundaries (what can and cannot be shared). Decisions are made as a group, often by generating a new, shared, conceptual framework. The predominant operating principle is one of integration.

Even if a team claims to be multidisciplinary, interdisciplinary, or transdisciplinary, it may have some characteristics of another structure depending on its size, composition, context, and stage of development. It is important to note that no value judgments are implied here: any structure may be appropriate and effective for a given setting, task, or group of people.

Foley (1990) pointed out that different team structures require different attitudes and expectations from their members. Recognizing that other professions have important contributions to make is essential to all team structures. For interdisciplinary and transdisciplinary teams, members must also be willing and able to work with others to make decisions jointly. Members of transdisciplinary teams additionally commit to teaching and learning from each other. As the amount of communication and interaction increases, more attention to the process of working together is needed.

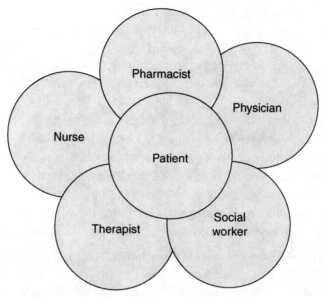

FIGURE 2.3 TRANSDISCIPLINARY TEAM STRUCTURE

VIGNETTE 2.2

Researchers from several departments form a group around topics of common interest. Enthusiasm for a new collaborative research project grows for a while but then slumps as the group works out the project details.

Several group members are disgruntled when two senior researchers submit a proposal without finalizing plans with the whole group. The senior researchers insist that they have the authority to act on behalf of the group. Someone suggests that the group spend a meeting discussing their expectations for participation, communication, and decision making.

What might happen if some people in a group assume they have an interdisciplinary team structure and others assume they have a multidisciplinary team structure?

Why might people from different departments of an organization have different expectations for team structure?

What might have happened if this group had discussed their expectations for communication and decision making at the outset?

Group Context

Groups exist within larger contexts. Workplace culture is the predominant context at the organizational level. Some groups are embedded firmly within one organization where all group members operate within the same workplace culture. Other groups cross organizations, or different parts or levels of a single organization, which may have different workplace cultures.

Differences in workplace culture can be significant barriers to teamwork. In practical terms, it may be difficult to find mutually satisfactory times and/ or places to meet. Less obvious are task-related issues, such as how much work each member can do, how quickly, and with what costs or benefits. The following are some characteristics of workplace culture that may differ among group members:

- Hours of work (e.g., 8-hour weekdays, 12-hour shifts, flexible time)
- Presence or absence of unions or employee associations
- Compensation practices (e.g., monthly salary, hourly rates, fee for service)
- Presence or absence of clerical and administrative support
- Workload expectations, including how overtime is managed
- Organizational styles (e.g., hierarchical, collegial)
- Predominant values (e.g., creativity, efficiency, accuracy, speed, flexibility)

In more general terms, individuals may differ substantially in the amount of control they have over their own schedules and activities. Incorrect assumptions about the workplace culture of other group members may lead to incorrect perceptions about the degree to which those members are committed to the group. Teamwork skills include both building awareness of differences in workplace cultures and checking out assumptions.

Even when a group is firmly embedded within one organizational culture, it may struggle if its style does not match the style of the larger organization. For example, group members may find it hard to work in a non-hierarchical way if the larger organization is hierarchical. In such cases, it is useful to have explicit discussions of these issues within the group and with relevant stakeholders from the larger organization.

I don't like having to work with people I'm incompatible with in terms of work ethics and values.

Authority and accountability also form part of the group context at the organizational level. Is the group self-directed or managed by others? Are the expectations and outcomes clear? What are the criteria for success? Who determines those criteria? What are the consequences for success or failure?

Finally, group context should also be considered at the systemic level: What is happening in the world outside the organization? Changes in economic, social, political, and technological domains can have significant effects on group functioning. Recognizing the impact of such systemic changes can help group members accommodate their goals to be more timely, realistic, or appropriate.

VIGNETTE 2.3

A diagnostic and treatment team for children with autism has frequent and prolonged conflict involving several team members. Everyone on the team agrees to engage the help of a third-party consultant experienced in conflict resolution.

In the course of their work with the consultant, team members realize that referrals to their services have more than doubled over the previous four years, reflecting the increasing awareness of autism in the larger community. Having identified that their workload has become unmanageable, they resolve to take several initiatives: 1) advocate for increased staffing, 2) streamline procedures, 3) set priorities, and 4) communicate with consumers of their services. Team members are relieved to be pulling in the same direction again.

How might an unmanageable workload lead to conflict among team members?

What are some advantages and disadvantages of having a third-party consultant work with a group in situations like this?

Group Development

Each working group has a life of its own. The group dynamics of a stable working group change over time, evolving along a predictable developmental course. Here is a brief description of these changes (adapted from Napier & Gershenfeld, 2004, pp. 403–411):

- At first, group members are typically polite, watchful, and cautious.
- As group members learn to trust one another, they move toward confrontation. Typically, group members work to balance conflict with harmony and sometimes reassessment.
- Members of successful working groups learn to resolve conflicts more quickly and easily over time. Limitations are acknowledged without blame.
- Members of dysfunctional working groups succumb to internal or external challenges that affect the group's emotional climate and/or its productivity.
- Finally, as a group moves toward adjournment or termination, members typically engage in reflection and evaluation and seek closure.

Various models of group development have been proposed over the past 60 years (Chidambaram & Bostrom, 1997; McCollom, 1990). The most famous is Tuckman's (1965) model of a sequence of four team stages: forming, storming, norming, and performing. (Rhymes make this model easy to remember.) A common feature of most models is that periods of conflict are expected. Knowing this can help those who dislike conflict learn to welcome it as a sign of increased trust and maturity in their working group.

EXERCISE 2.3

Look up and study Tuckman's model of the stages of group development[1] and then answer the following questions:

What do the terms forming, storming, norming, *and* performing *mean?*

_____

_____

_____

What kind of groups did Tuckman analyze for his model of team stages?

_____

_____

_____

What are the limitations of a successive stage model?

_____

_____

_____

In most long-term groups, turnover is inevitable. When membership changes in a group, the group reverts to an earlier stage of development. The balance of task and group maintenance (discussed in chapter 3) shifts for a time as the newcomer and the established group members accommodate one another. Long-term groups often follow a generational paradigm in which old members are gradually replaced by new ones. In this paradigm, group norms persist over several generations, although arbitrary norms decay faster. Such groups often develop leadership systems based on seniority and become more proficient at carrying out tasks with time. It is incumbent on leaders of long-term groups to manage turnover by orienting newcomers and facilitating their integration into the group.

Turnover in working groups is often seen as negative, but it may be neutral or may even have positive effects. Levine and Choi (2004, pp. 153–176) reviewed research on the cost-benefit ratio related to personnel turnover and identified several factors:

- **Group structure:** Turnover is negative for more interactive groups.
- **Task difficulty:** Turnover is negative for more routine tasks.
- **Time course:** Increasing or unpredictable rates of turnover have a negative effect.
- **Membership dynamics:** Turnover is negative for more central group members.

While turnover may be costly, newcomers may also enhance group performance by introducing innovations and generating ideas. Research has shown that groups with changing membership are more creative than more stable groups. A positive newcomer effect is more likely when groups are open to new members, understaffed, in an early stage of development, and/or performing poorly (Levine, Choi, & Moreland, 2003).

In summary, group dynamics are complex and changeable. While no single member can fully appreciate all the factors that contribute to how a group is working at any given time, awareness of how the group's size, composition, structure, context, and development contribute to the dynamics is important. These factors account for why people show different attitudes and aspects of their personality in different groups and at different times.

Applying the Framework

In this chapter, we have delineated the attitudes, skills, and knowledge that constitute the domain of teamwork competencies for interprofessional collaboration. The three vignettes in this chapter illustrate how these teamwork competencies apply to different levels of context: interpersonal, organizational, and systemic (see Table 2.1). Vignette 2.1 illustrates teamwork issues at the interpersonal level by highlighting the importance of demonstrating respect consistently. Vignette 2.2 illustrates teamwork issues at the organizational level by pointing out the need for clarity about a group's structure and process. Vignette 2.3 illustrates teamwork issues at the systemic level by showing how increased workloads stemming from population changes can lead to a siege mentality in a group.

TABLE 2.1 FRAMEWORK FOR TEAMWORK

	INTERPERSONAL	ORGANIZATIONAL	SYSTEMIC
Teamwork	Respect	Group structure	Population changes

EXERCISE 2.4

Reflect on your own experiences of teamwork and then answer the following questions:

What keywords can you add to the cells in the framework in Table 2.1 that pertain to each of your stories?

_____

_____

_____

How might this framework inform your analysis of these stories?

_____

_____

_____

It is evident that these three levels of context operate simultaneously and no situation can be reduced to only one contextual level or competency domain. Skilled collaborators keep all domains and levels in mind while focusing on one or two cells of the framework to enhance their understanding of a specific situation. By clarifying your attitudes toward working with others, honing your interpersonal skills, and expanding your knowledge about group dynamics, you can infuse your collaborative work with energy and optimism. You can then look forward to meetings like the one described at the beginning of this chapter: filled with energy, optimism, humor, and respect; where group members value the time they spend together and use that time well.

NOTES

1 For a useful explanation and critique of Tuckman's model of team stages, see the entry in the online encyclopedia of informal education by Smith (2005) titled "Bruce W. Tuckman – Forming, storming, norming and performing in groups": www.infed.org/mobi /bruce-w-tuckman-forming-storming-norming-and-performing-in-groups/

3

Leadership

Imagine a group that identifies goals and develops plans in the best interests of its stakeholders. Everyone contributes and takes ownership for managing conflict and solving problems. There are no hidden agendas, no hurt feelings . . .

AFTER READING THIS CHAPTER, YOU WILL BE ABLE TO DO THE FOLLOWING:

- Distinguish between different *leadership roles*
- Contrast *classical and shared leadership*
- Identify group values and norms for *participatory decision making*
- Recognize *leadership behavior* that accomplishes group tasks and builds and maintains the group
- Explain the *benefits and costs of conflict*
- Appreciate different styles of *conflict management*
- *Apply the framework* to understand challenges in leadership

Just as the paradox of teamwork is that it is an individual skill, the paradox of leadership in collaborative settings is that it is a shared skill. We often think of a group leader as one person in a position of authority, but in collaborative work, any group member may step into a leadership role when needed. Effective leaders show initiative, judgment, sensitivity, and good timing; they also understand the principles of participatory decision making and conflict resolution. Ultimately, leaders are responsible for maintaining group cohesiveness and achieving the group's goals. Collaborative work succeeds best when every participant's leadership skills are used.

Leadership Roles

Leadership overlaps with official roles, including those of manager and facilitator. Many people assume that leaders are those in positions of authority: those at or near the top of an organizational chart. However, leaders without officially sanctioned authority often emerge spontaneously within an organization or group. Professionals who understand the nuances of these different roles are better prepared to decide when to lead, and when and whom to follow.

While managers may be leaders, leadership is not inherent to the role of manager. In business, including the business of healthcare, managers are responsible for day-to-day operations. Leadership, on the other hand, is demonstrated by one who has a vision — a mental picture of a desired future state — and who gets others to understand and believe in that vision. People work for managers; people follow leaders (Bennis & Nanus, 1997, pp. 200–203).

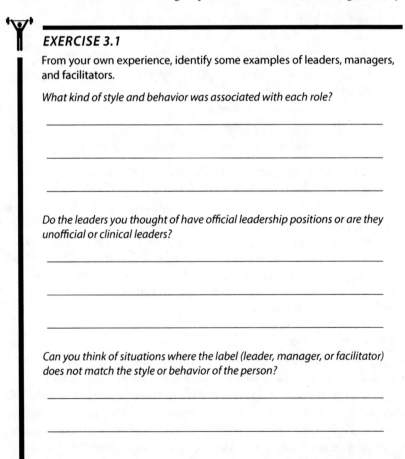

Sometimes it's not clear what everyone's roles are so it's hard to know who is responsible for what.

Facilitation is a specific kind of leadership characterized by neutrality. A facilitator focuses on both the content and process of group discussions and decisions. While managers are typically accountable to their superiors, facilitators are accountable to all the members of a group and have no decision-making authority.

EXERCISE 3.1

From your own experience, identify some examples of leaders, managers, and facilitators.

What kind of style and behavior was associated with each role?

_____

_____

_____

Do the leaders you thought of have official leadership positions or are they unofficial or clinical leaders?

_____

_____

_____

Can you think of situations where the label (leader, manager, or facilitator) does not match the style or behavior of the person?

_____

_____

_____

We often think of leadership as something shown by one individual, but leaders are successful only insofar as followers agree to work toward the same vision. In collaborative groups especially, leadership is shared. The concept of shared leadership — also called distributed, team, inclusive, or democratic leadership — has emerged to account for the practice of leadership within groups (Nemerowicz & Rosi, 1997; Spillane, 2005). Admittedly, this is a complex area discussed and debated in detail by scholars of administration and leadership in education, business, and healthcare. The ideas presented here introduce the concept of shared leadership, with a focus on practical application.

Classical and Shared Leadership

Classical models of leadership are associated with charisma, vision, power, and authority (Doyle & Smith, 2001a). In the workplace, leaders traditionally influence subordinates in a vertical relationship with an emphasis on control or oversight (Pearce & Conger, 2003). As shown in Table 3.1, classical leaders are established by position or authority, use formal lines of communication, and provide solutions to problems. In a classical model of leadership, leaders are thought to differ from those they lead in some way, such as character, skill, or motivation. Classical leaders may control information as a source of power and are subject to the corrupting influences of power.

TABLE 3.1 CLASSICAL LEADERSHIP COMPARED WITH SHARED LEADERSHIP

CLASSICAL LEADERSHIP	SHARED LEADERSHIP
Leader established by position in a hierarchy	Leaders identified by the quality of their interactions
Evaluated by how the leader solves problems	Evaluated by how people work together
Group members expect the leader to provide answers or solutions	Group members take ownership for problems, seek common good
Leader differs from others in character, skill, or motivation	Leadership based on teachable/learnable attributes of curiosity, empathy, creativity, and cooperativeness
Formal communication style	Informal communication style with an emphasis on listening
Information retained and controlled as a source of power	Information freely sought and shared
May use secrecy, deception, or payoffs	Relies on democratic process, honesty, and shared ethics

Source: Adapted from M. E. Doyle & M. K. Smith (2001b). Shared leadership. *The encyclopedia of informal education*; G. Nemerowicz & E. Rosi (1997). *Education for leadership and social responsibility*. London, UK: Falmer Press, p. 16.

The concept of shared leadership is rooted in advances in the fields of organizational behavior and psychology during the 20th century (Pearce & Conger, 2003). It is characterized by a horizontal relationship among peers who create conditions for collective learning (Fletcher & Käufer, 2003). Shared leadership has been defined as "a dynamic, interactive influence process among individuals in groups for which the objective is to lead one another to the achievement of group or organizational goals or both" (Pearce & Conger, 2003, p. 1). In this model, leaders are identified by the quality of their interactions and evaluated by how well the group is working (see Table 3.1). All group members take ownership for problem solving and contribute to the process of leadership by pursuing the common good through diversity. Generally, communication is informal, with an emphasis on listening, seeking, and sharing information. Power is distributed among group members, though not necessarily equally. This distribution of power leads to an emphasis on ethics, honesty, and the democratic process in decision making.

EXERCISE 3.2

Consider how the power of leadership can lead to an abuse of power, using an example from your own experience or from history, politics, sports, or entertainment.

What problems did this abuse of power lead to?

_____

_____

_____

How did other people limit or counteract this abuse of power?

_____

_____

_____

Classical leaders may not welcome leadership by other group members. Confusion and conflict may erupt when group members challenge classical leaders. There is also a cost, however, to remaining silent about strong feelings or beliefs. As Avery points out, "going along" leads to one of two outcomes:

"entire groups going where no member wants to go, [or] people hanging out together with low commitment, low energy, low performance, resentment, and low esteem" (2001, p. 33). Authority relationships are, in the end, simply agreements between people. Participants in collaboration always retain their personal power and should treat every action and decision as something they consent to; if not, they may choose to decline that relationship (pp. 32–33).

Some people don't have the ability to be a team player. It's their way or the highway.

The extent to which a shared leadership model is adopted by a group depends to some extent on the structure of the group. For example, transdisciplinary team members by definition adopt a shared leadership model as they share expertise and learn from one another. In contrast, members of some multidisciplinary teams or administrative groups may agree to more traditional models of leadership. Groups with members who share the same mental model of group structure and leadership waste less time on power struggles and proceed more efficiently toward their goals.

Participatory Decision Making

Participatory decision making is beneficial when there is a distribution of knowledge among members of the group and there is a need for high-quality decisions that all can accept (Vroom, 2000). In healthcare, such situations arise when patient needs and problems are multiple, complex, and/or overlap professional boundaries (Heinemann et al., 1999). Interprofessional collaboration in healthcare requires that all professionals have a shared understanding of the principles of participatory decision making. In addition, participatory decision making that includes the patient and/or family members is fundamental to patient- and family-centered care.

Not everyone's opinions are considered.

Kaner (2007, pp. 24–29) identified four core values of participatory decision making:

- **Full participation:** Members take risks to share ideas with each other, even when some ideas are not yet fully developed. Members encourage each other to speak up rather than remaining quiet and/or talking outside the meeting.
- **Mutual understanding:** Members listen to each other's ideas actively and put effort into seeing multiple perspectives. When difficult issues are addressed by the group, there is recognition of diversity among the

group and the legitimacy of the needs and goals of each member. Opposing views can co-exist: they are not seen as conflict that must be resolved or suppressed.

- **Inclusive solutions:** Members persist in generating innovative solutions that are understood by and work for all affected, rather than expecting some to acquiesce to persuasion.
- **Shared responsibility:** Members readily accept responsibility for the decision-making process and for the outcomes of their decisions.

Kaner pointed out that participatory decision making generates solutions

> whose range and vision are expanded to take advantage
> of the truth held not only by the quick, the articulate, the
> influential, and the powerful, but also of the truth held by
> those who are shy or disenfranchised or who think at a
> slower pace. (p. 24)

When group members adopt these values, they ensure that the process of decision making supports collaborative and/or patient- and family-centered care.

VIGNETTE 3.1

Frank, a 56-year-old man, attends his annual diabetic clinic appointment. His interdisciplinary team includes a nurse, a physician, a dietitian, and a social worker. After some preliminary discussion, the dialogue continues as follows:

Dietitian: Frank, I notice that your diet is somewhat restricted.

Physician: And his sugars aren't in the target range.

Frank: Yeah.

Nurse: I have completed the care plan. Should we increase his insulin?

Physician: Yes, let's increase it by 10%.

Dietitian: So Frank, I think we should spend some time figuring out what's going on with your food and cooking.

Frank: Okay.

Nurse: When should we see him again?

Physician: Annually.

How do these team members support inclusiveness?

Do they exclude anyone? How?

Who is sharing responsibility for the outcome of this meeting?

What actions could team members take to promote full participation and mutual understanding?

Decision rules are the single most important element of participatory decision making. Without explicit agreement on decision rules, group members may not even be sure when or if a decision has been made (Kaner, 2007, pp. 266–267). Groups that have clarity on how they make decisions are more likely to engage the commitment of all group members to those decisions. Decision rules do not have to be rigid: groups may use different rules for different situations. Kaner reviewed the use of different decision rules for high-stakes and low-stakes decisions (pp. 270–274):

> You need to give up some ideas that you like in order to go with the group's ideas.

- **Unanimous agreement** is the best option when the stakes are high and/or when support by a minority viewpoint is essential. Because unanimous agreement requires listening, persistence, and reconciling different perspectives, it often takes more time than the other decision rules. Note that unanimous agreement differs from a consensus based on compromise in which people agree to something that they don't fully support.
- **Majority vote** can work for low-stakes decisions when expedience is more important than quality. For high-stakes decisions, the process of voting may take on an adversarial quality based on political alliances rather than the merits of a proposal. Using secret ballots can increase the likelihood that votes are based on the merits of the proposal.
- **Person-in-charge decides after discussion** is justifiable for high-stakes decisions, if the discussion has been open and inclusive. To ensure open and inclusive discussion, groups may choose to meet separately from the person-in-charge or to use procedures that encourage "devil's advocate" thinking. Since there is less risk associated with low-stakes decisions, this decision rule produces similar results for low-risk decisions as unanimous agreement and majority vote.
- **Flip-a-coin** includes any arbitrary method such as drawing straws; obviously, it would not be appropriate for a high-stakes decision. When the stakes are low, arbitrary methods reduce participation and discussion, which may be desirable in some cases (such as deciding where to go for lunch).
- **Person-in-charge decides without discussion** is appropriate in the midst of a crisis. However, this decision rule is risky for high-stakes decisions because of the potential for blind spots on the part of the person-in-charge or for sabotaging by others in the group. When the stakes are low, the risks associated with bad decisions are lower as well.

Kaner noted that each decision rule "has a different effect on group behavior. Individual group members adjust the quantity and quality of their participation depending on how they think their behavior will influence the decision" (p. 274). For this reason, good leadership entails judgment in choosing the right decision rule for the situation.

Ethical standards are important to decision making in healthcare and add additional complexity. While all professionals should be competent to work through ethical dilemmas according to their own standards, it is often helpful to consult with others as part of this process. By so doing, group members are more likely to share ownership of the resolution of ethical dilemmas and will recognize those (likely rare) instances where different professionals' ethical standards conflict.

Leadership Behavior

The more leadership is shared and the greater the degree of interaction and joint decision making, the more group members need to attend to the process of working together. To understand how shared leadership works, leadership behavior in groups must be examined at a micro-level. A time-honored list of shared leadership roles assumed by group members was developed by Benne and Sheats (1948) and has been summarized and republished repeatedly (Bass, 1990; Harnack, Fest, & Jones, 1977). An essential feature of this list is that shared leadership behavior falls within one of two distinct categories: group task and group building/maintenance. In this section, we present our adaptation of this classic list.

Group Task Behavior

The following actions serve to further the group toward its tasks or goals:

- **Initiating:** proposing goals, setting agendas, defining problems, suggesting solutions, developing plans
- **Seeking information:** asking for facts, information, opinions, ideas, and feelings
- **Giving information:** offering facts, information, opinions, ideas, and feelings
- **Clarifying and elaborating:** interpreting ideas, clearing up confusions, defining terms, indicating alternatives, giving examples
- **Summarizing:** restating or pulling together related ideas
- **Consensus testing:** offering a conclusion to see if the group agrees

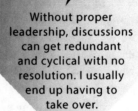

Without proper leadership, discussions can get redundant and cyclical with no resolution. I usually end up having to take over.

- **Evaluating:** examining the feasibility and rightness of ideas, evaluating alternatives, comparing group decisions with group standards and goals
- **Recording:** ensuring that a written record is made of group ideas, decisions, and plans

Group Building and Maintenance Behavior

The following actions serve to develop and maintain the group:

- **Harmonizing:** reconciling disagreements, reducing tension (by using humor, suggesting breaks, offering fun approaches to work)
- **Gatekeeping and trust building:** encouraging everyone to participate, demonstrating acceptance and openness to the ideas of others, encouraging individuality, promoting open discussion of conflicts
- **Supporting and encouraging:** being friendly, warm, and responsive (in speech, gesture, facial expression), giving recognition for contributions
- **Compromising:** admitting error, shifting position in response to new insights
- **Coordinating and regulating:** drawing together activities of members or subgroups, influencing the direction and tempo of the group's work

Benne and Sheats (1948) originally conceptualized these task and group-maintenance behavior categories as roles that individual group members take on. We propose that it is more useful to think of these behavior categories as actions that any group member may perform. Certainly, individuals have a habitual repertoire, a subset of actions that they use frequently. For example, some of us are more task-focused and others orient more to group maintenance. Regardless, we are all capable of both kinds of leadership. In a shared leadership environment, any member of the group may demonstrate any leadership behavior as the need arises. It is important to recognize that a balance of both task and group-maintenance leadership is required for groups to achieve their goals (Bass, 1990, pp. 473–510). In the section on conflict management later in this chapter, we provide an example of why and how to shift focus from task to group maintenance.

Benne and Sheats (1948) also identified that members of groups may engage in behavior that serves their individual needs rather than the needs of the group. Interestingly, they point out that a high incidence of such individual-centered behavior calls for self-diagnosis by the group. For example, groups with a lot of individual-centered behavior may have an inadequately defined task; a low level of group maturity, discipline, or morale; or a prevalence of authoritarian or laissez-faire attitudes toward the group. We have adapted Benne and Sheats's description of individual-centered behavior and called it group-hindering behavior.

EXERCISE 3.3

Obtain permission from a working group to observe a meeting. Print off the checklist in Appendix B and use it to observe the interactions of members of this group.

What types of task-oriented behavior did you observe?

_____

_____

_____

What types of group maintenance behavior did you observe?

_____

_____

_____

How did the group respond to these actions?

_____

_____

_____

What types of behavior do you typically use yourself?

_____

_____

_____

Are there some types of behavior that you don't often use that you would like to try in your next working group meeting?

_____

_____

_____

Group-Hindering Behavior

The following actions serve the personal needs of the individual without regard for the group's task achievement or maintenance needs:

- **Blocking:** arguing, resisting, disagreeing in a way that interferes with group progress
- **Out of field:** withdrawing from discussion, daydreaming, whispering to others
- **Intimidating:** expressing disapproval of others, joking aggressively
- **Digressing:** getting off the subject, making a long rambling speech
- **Recognition seeking:** calling attention to oneself by boasting, appealing for sympathy, displaying unusual nonverbal behavior

Any of us may engage, from time to time, in behavior related to our personal needs at the expense of the group. In a mature group, hindering functions are recognized and addressed with respect, sensitivity, and even humor, if appropriate. Effective leaders recognize when they themselves are engaging in hindering actions and take steps to change their behavior or remedy the situation. Often, reflecting on the nature of the hindering behavior can give clues about what is needed by the group; for example, clarification of group norms or goals, change of pace, or checking out assumptions.

Benefits and Costs of Conflict

Conflict can be constructive and energizing, or it can be destructive and divisive. In chapter 2, we learned that conflict is inevitable when groups of individuals with diverse viewpoints join together to fashion meanings, establish goals, define purposes, clarify roles, and take action. Conflict is productive when it leads to new understandings and creative solutions. It is destructive when it becomes personal, chronic, or hidden. Understanding conflict and keeping conflict productive are important functions of leadership.

Simple opposition does not necessarily result in conflict. Opposition is defined as resistance or dissent in action or argument. Some of the most creative ideas arise from the synergy of opposition. In contrast, conflict is a sharp collision of interests, ideas, or principles resulting in emotional disturbance. This emotional component characterizes interpersonal conflict in collaboration.

Elias Porter, a social psychologist, developed a framework to understand interpersonal conflict called Relationship Awareness Theory (Porter, 1996). According to this theory, each of us has a motivational value system that underpins all of our relationship behavior. We act to get things done, but also to be congruent with our values — to confirm our self-worth. Conflict is an internal experience that occurs when a person perceives his or her sense of self-worth to be threatened. Because different people have different sets of values, they go into conflict at different times and for different reasons. One benefit of conflict is that we learn what is important to others when we observe that they are in conflict.

People vary in how they show conflict. For some, obvious changes in behavior signal that they are experiencing conflict. This can be uncomfortable for others present who witness the changes. Others exhibit minimal outward change when they enter conflict, so that their colleagues may not recognize that they are in conflict or understand the degree of conflict they are experiencing. Individuals also vary in self-awareness. Some know immediately that they are in conflict, while others require time to process their feelings. The expression of conflict is also influenced by power differentials, relationship history, age, gender, and culture.

> I don't like collaborating because conflicts develop that don't ever get resolved.

EXERCISE 3.4

Explore the website[1] of Personal Strengths Publishing (2015) to learn about five keys to having a nice conflict and then answer the following questions:

What are some of the costs of conflict?

_____

_____

_____

How can one anticipate and prevent conflict?

_____

_____

_____

Conflicts about goals or purpose are necessary and must be managed for the group to make progress. For example, a group of health professionals may argue about whether their goal is one of disease management or one of disease prevention. Unnecessary conflict, on the other hand, arises from clashes in relating styles or misunderstandings about others' values. For example, a group that has agreed to work on disease prevention may experience conflict when planning how to proceed: some individuals may value acting decisively, rolling out a program immediately, while others may value acting judiciously, collecting more data before going public. When group members learn to recognize each other's underlying values, they can respectfully discuss ideas without threatening each other's self-worth, thus preventing needless conflict.

Relationship Awareness Theory also posits that conflict proceeds through three distinct stages (Porter, 1996). Initially, individuals in conflict work to preserve their relationships with others, to solve the problem, and to maintain their own core values. If conflict deepens, individuals may disconnect from their relationships with others while still working to solve the problem and maintain their core values. In the last stage, even the problem is abandoned — self-preservation is all that matters. Effective leaders recognize interpersonal conflict early and work to prevent it from deepening.

VIGNETTE 3.2

An internal medicine department has broadened representation at departmental meetings to improve communication between health professionals and hospital administration. A situation has arisen that impacts patient safety and requires new resources as well as a change in process.

While some clinicians are describing the problem and its implications, a few others respond with sarcastic comments and hint that the concern is not that significant. Those who are concerned continue to justify their reasons even more energetically with examples. A senior administrator rolls his eyes and other group members begin to check email. Gradually, discussion ceases and no solution emerges.

Later, the concerned clinicians discuss the situation in the hallway. They feel the situation is unresolved. They worry that if they continue to express their concerns without the support of the rest of their group, they will be viewed as troublemakers by administration.

What is the conflict? How do we know there is conflict?

What stage of conflict might each person be experiencing?

Is this conflict necessary or unnecessary?

What suggestions would you have for this group?

Conflict Management

Conflict is part of group process and is often necessary for deeper under-standing and better problem solving, but conflict does make most people uncomfortable. Furthermore, as people feel threatened, frustrated, confused, or impatient, they become more emotional and may be less courteous or respectful. Such heightened emotions may be a symptom that the conflict is moving into the second stage. Leadership is required to get through the rough spots for a truly collaborative, win–win outcome.

In the influential *Handbook of Industrial and Organizational Psychology*, Kenneth Thomas published a taxonomy of conflict management (1976; see also Thomas, 1992). This taxonomy has five conflict-handling styles that vary along a dimension of assertiveness (attempting to satisfy one's own concerns) and a second dimension of cooperativeness (attempting to satisfy others' concerns):

- **Competing:** high assertiveness, low cooperativeness (The goal is to win.)
- **Avoiding:** low assertiveness, low cooperativeness (The goal is to delay.)
- **Accommodating:** low assertiveness, high cooperation (The goal is to yield.)
- **Compromising:** mid-assertiveness, mid-cooperation (The goal is to find a middle ground.)
- **Collaborating:** high assertiveness, high cooperation (The goal is to find a win–win solution.)

Over the years, this taxonomy has earned a great deal of empirical support and has generated valid psychometric measures of people's habitual approach to conflict (Thomas, 1992).

While Thomas originally advocated for collaboration as the ideal style of conflict management, he later acknowledged that further refinement of his conceptualization was required to account for research on the functionality of conflict-handling styles (Thomas, 1992). Specifically, he added two new dimensions: choice of beneficiary and time frame. Choice of beneficiary may be partisan (one of the parties involved), joint-welfare (both parties), or sys-temic (the larger system of which parties are members). Time frame may be short term or long term. For short-term or partisan goals, individuals may be pragmatic in their style of conflict management. For example, "one does not try collaboration if there are competitive incentives and procedures, if the parties have insufficient problem-solving skills, if the time is too short, and if neither party trusts the other" (Thomas, 1992, p. 271). In contrast, collaboration is essential for long-term goals that relate to changing the sys-tem: to address those structural variables that result in poor outcomes.

Thomas's taxonomy of conflict styles is useful for understanding common ways of managing conflict and their effect on both group maintenance and task accomplishment. Of course, how someone manages conflict depends on the circumstances, including the group, the issue, and the context. As well, people may manage conflict differently at different stages of the conflict process. For example, someone who is task-oriented might initially compete and then change to compromising as other points of view are understood, while someone who is more oriented to group maintenance might initially accommodate but switch to avoiding as conflict deepens. Most of us have a preferred or habitual response to conflict. It can be helpful to reflect on our habits or knee-jerk responses. Training in conflict management often involves helping people to assess a situation and choose the most appropriate conflict style for that situation, rather than relying on their habitual style.

EXERCISE 3.5

The Thomas-Kilmann Conflict Mode Instrument (Thomas & Kilmann, 2007) is a self-assessment tool that indicates what conflict modes a person may be overusing or underusing. Study their website[2] and the sample report and then answer the following questions:

What might you learn about yourself from completing this instrument?

_____

_____

_____

Do the authors of this instrument feel that there is one best way to handle conflict?

_____

_____

_____

What are some signs of overuse of a collaborative style of conflict resolution?

_____

_____

_____

Recent research has illuminated how conflict styles vary for men and women at different levels of an organization. Thomas, Fann Thomas, and Schaubhut (2008) analyzed the conflict styles of a stratified random sample drawn from a national database. This sample included 200 men and 200 women at each of six organizational levels: entry level, non-supervisory, supervisor, management, executive, and top executive. They found a linear increase for assertive styles (collaborating and competing) at progressively higher organizational levels, while unassertive styles (accommodating and avoiding) decreased. Compromising, the most widely used conflict style, was highest at the four middle organizational levels and lowest at the entry and top executive levels. Interestingly, men scored significantly higher than women did on competing at all organizational levels. This research illustrates how a conflict style for any given situation is related to many factors: personal, organizational, and systemic.

VIGNETTE 3.3

A speech-language pathologist (SLP) has begun seeing Mrs. Albert, an 88-year-old woman who has had a stroke. During the SLP's intake assessment, he notes that Mrs. Albert has both speech and swallowing issues. In this outpatient clinic, occupational therapy (OT) works with swallowing disorders, which are within the scope of practice of both professions. Here is part of the conversation between the SLP and the OT:

SLP: Mrs. Albert is coming back in next week so that I can finish my initial assessment and make a plan for therapy. She definitely has speech issues, but I've also observed some swallowing concerns. Instead of you having to schedule sessions with her too, I thought I could work on the swallowing concerns as well.

OT: Oh, I hadn't heard about Mrs. Albert.

SLP: Well, I just got the referral and only started her diagnostic assessment today. I know she's going to need therapy for speech and for swallowing. If you want to see her too, that's fine. I can ask her referring physician to set that up. But I was thinking that it'd be easier for all of us to do it this way.

OT: Um. Fine. (The OT turns and walks away briskly and goes to their manager to complain about the SLP taking away her clients.)

What is the conflict?

Which conflict-handling styles are exhibited?

What suggestions would you have for resolving this conflict?

Regardless of conflict style, one useful strategy to manage conflict in a group is to shift the focus from task to group maintenance. To make this shift, Kaner (2007, p. 143) suggested the following steps:

- Describe the predicament supported by your observations: "We keep discussing something we've already decided. Two people have raised this issue even though we've moved on to another topic."
- Obtain agreement to shift focus: "I propose that we step back from the situation for a moment to learn more about what's going on. I have an idea for a simple way to do this, if you all agree."
- When agreement is obtained, pose a question that helps the group focus on their process: "Does anyone have any thoughts about how we are working together?"
- After a few responses, pose a more specific question: "What might be preventing us from working together more effectively?"
- When group members appear ready to return to the original discussion, prepare for the shift: "Before we return to our (task/topic), are there any further comments about what we've just been talking about?"

When groups are stuck, goofy, fragmented, or argumentative, changing focus from task to group maintenance can help group members regain their equilibrium.

Open discussion can be the least effective format for managing conflict because of the pressure to speak articulately and persuasively. Kaner (2007, p. 142) offered these suggestions when open discussion becomes dysfunctional:

- Switch to brainstorming.
- Break into small groups.
- Switch to a structured go-around.
- Encourage more people to participate in the discussion.
- Switch to individual writing.

When group members agree to one of these alternatives to open discussion, they manage conflict by applying the principles of participatory decision making. Changing the pattern of interaction in this way can also boost the energy of the group and renew the commitment of its members.

EXERCISE 3.6

While brainstorming is commonly used, not everyone knows how to run a brainstorming session well. The website for TEDBlog[3] has an entry on how to run a brainstorm for introverts (and extroverts too) (McClure, 2014). Study the blog and then answer the following questions:

Why might some people cringe when faced with a brainstorming session?

_____

_____

_____

What attitudes and behaviors of the brainstorm leader promote creativity and confidence in all group members?

_____

_____

_____

Applying the Framework

In this chapter, we have delineated the values, attitudes, skills, and knowledge that constitute the domain of leadership competencies for interprofessional collaboration. The three vignettes in this chapter illustrate how these leadership competencies apply to different levels of context: interpersonal, organizational, and systemic (see Table 3.2). Vignette 3.1 illustrates how leadership is needed at the interpersonal level to ensure full participation in decision making. Vignette 3.2 illustrates how leadership is needed at the organizational level to manage conflict about resources and procedures. Vignette 3.3 illustrates leadership issues at the systemic level by showing how overlapping scopes of practice can lead to conflict about professional roles and relationships.

TABLE 3.2 FRAMEWORK FOR LEADERSHIP

	INTERPERSONAL	ORGANIZATIONAL	SYSTEMIC
Leadership	Participatory decision making	Conflict about resources and procedures	Conflict about scope of practice

EXERCISE 3.7

Reflect on your own experiences of leadership and then answer the following questions:

What keywords can you add to the cells in the framework in Table 3.2 that pertain to each of your stories?

_____

_____

_____

How might this framework inform your analysis of these stories?

_____

_____

_____

Leadership is an amorphous concept that dominates the writing of business, management, and teamwork gurus. In this chapter, we have identified how all members of a collaborative group can show leadership, even though they may not be officially recognized leaders. By clarifying your values and beliefs, understanding the principles of participatory decision making, developing task-focused and group maintenance skills, and increasing your repertoire of conflict management styles, you can contribute to high-performing groups. The group described at the beginning of this chapter is the goal for all working groups: one that identifies goals and develops plans in the best interests of its stakeholders; where everyone contributes and takes ownership for managing conflict and solving problems with no hidden agendas or hurt feelings.

NOTES

1 www.personalstrengths.ca/relationship-awareness/managing-conflict/
2 www.kilmanndiagnostics.com/catalog/thomas-kilmann-conflict-mode-instrument
3 http://blog.ted.com/how-to-run-a-brainstorm-for-introverts-and-extroverts-too/

4

Communication

Imagine an easy and worry-free discussion with your team, where you have confidence that the messages sent are the ones intended to be sent and that those listening receive those messages in the way they were intended. There is no second-guessing yourself or finding out later that people misunderstood . . .

AFTER READING THIS CHAPTER, YOU WILL BE ABLE TO DO THE FOLLOWING:

- Appreciate how *communication in small groups* differs from dyadic communication
- Identify ways to be clear and forthright in *face-to-face communication* using nonverbal signals and spoken language
- Describe how to share responsibility for clear communication by *active listening*
- Be conscious of the advantages and disadvantages of *asynchronous communication*, especially writing and reading
- Explain how *informal communication* supports interprofessional collaboration
- Recognize the role that *self-awareness* plays in communication, especially for stereotyping and hidden agendas
- Choose *communication tools* to strengthen interprofessional collaboration
- *Apply the framework* to understand challenges in communication

Like teamwork and leadership, communication for collaboration has its paradox: communication is widely endorsed as the most important component of effective collaboration (Baerg et al., 2012), but health professionals and students may have negative attitudes toward communication training (Rees & Garrud, 2001; Rees, Sheard, & McPherson, 2002). Communication has been identified as the source of both positive and negative collaboration experiences (Hartrick Doane, Stajduhar, Causton, Bidgood, & Cox, 2012). Good communication contributes to efficient and effective outcomes and fosters a sense of well-being within the team (Wertheimer et al., 2008). In contrast, poor communication leads to errors, unsatisfactory patient care, and poor team morale (Farahani, Sahragard, Caroll, & Mohammadi, 2011). To communicate for collaboration, you need to understand the challenges of communicating in small groups, to express yourself clearly, to listen and read actively, and to be aware of your own goals and biases.

Communication in Small Groups

Communication is the act of exchanging information through a shared system of signs: words, gestures, and other behaviors. We receive, process, and transmit information to effect change. Communication is not perfect: signs used by a sender are not complete representations of the sender's intent, and the interpretation of those signs by the receiver does not map precisely onto the intention of the sender. As Chandler put it, "Meaning is not 'transmitted' to us — we actively create it according to a complex interplay of codes or conventions of which we are normally unaware" (2007, p. 11). As the number of communicators increases, so does the potential for variations in created meaning.

Most health professional education programs teach skills for dyadic (one-to-one) communication with patients. These skills may include any or all of the following: building rapport, showing empathy, avoiding stereotyping, gathering information by asking open questions, active listening (e.g., for emotions, beliefs, attributions, expectations), checking on patient understanding, clarifying, managing the interview, and avoiding jargon (Cegala & Lenzmeier Broz, 2002; Chant, Jenkinson, Randle, Russell, & Webb, 2002; Duffy, Gordon, Whelan, Cole-Kelly, & Frankel, 2004). All of these skills allow both partners in dyadic communication to ensure that the meaning they are making is compatible. Within dyads, it is a relatively straightforward process to verify how messages have been received and to repair failures in communication.

To appreciate how communication in small groups differs from dyadic communication, consider the following two examples. The first example is of a simple dyadic exchange: person A speaks and person B responds (see Figure 4.1). Within this one-directional conversational turn, there are four potential meanings: A's intended meaning, B's understanding of what A says, B's intended meaning, and A's understanding of what B says. In the second example, four individuals have similar one-directional conversational turns with each other (see Figure 4.2). This set of six turns

Information gets lost in multiple communications.

(AB, AC, AD, BC, BD, and CD), for which each turn has four potential meanings, yields 24 potential meanings. In addition, those in the group not directly involved in the conversational turn also construct meaning of what they hear. For example, C and D construct meanings of what A and B say to each other, adding another four potential meanings per turn, producing 24 additional meanings. Thus, there are in total 48 potential meanings among four group

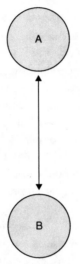

FIGURE 4.1 CONVERSATIONAL TURN BETWEEN TWO PEOPLE

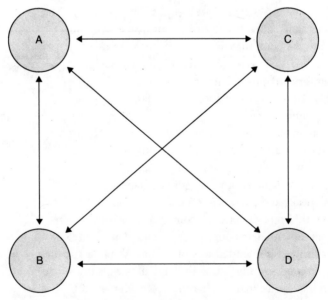

FIGURE 4.2 CONVERSATIONAL TURNS IN A GROUP OF FOUR PEOPLE

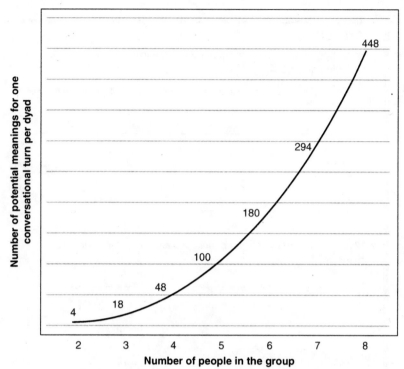

FIGURE 4.3 POTENTIAL MEANINGS AS A FUNCTION OF GROUP SIZE

members over six conversational turns. Figure 4.3 shows how the number of potential meanings increases in a curvilinear relationship as group size increases.

Of course, real conversations in small groups are more fluid, chaotic, and imbalanced than those of the contrived example described above. Nevertheless, this way of considering the number of potential meanings in a conversation makes it clear why there is such a risk for misunderstandings in groups. Furthermore, small groups do not allow for easy repair of communication problems, since people may refrain from checking assumptions or asking for clarification because of internal inhibitions (e.g., lack of confidence) or external constraints (e.g., time pressures). These observations are supported by research that shows that trust and cooperation are established more easily in dyads than in small groups regardless of the medium of communication (face-to-face vs. computer-based text chat) (Lev-On, Chavez, & Bicchieri, 2010). To meet the inherent challenges of small-group communication, we must take care to send messages effectively and to listen actively.

EXERCISE 4.1

Reflecting on your own communication strengths and style, answer the following questions:

How comfortable are you speaking in a dyad? In a small group? In a large group?

_____

_____

_____

What characteristics of a group make you feel more or less comfortable speaking?

_____

_____

_____

Do you tend to talk a lot in groups? If so, what signals tell you that you need to step back and let others talk?

_____

_____

_____

Are you generally quiet in groups? If so, what signals tell you that you need to step up and share your thoughts or questions?

_____

_____

_____

Face-to-Face Communication

Skilled communicators in small groups pay attention to all aspects of the complex process of communication. They ensure that their nonverbal signals are congruent with their spoken words. They choose the most apt words, phrases, and overall structure when speaking and writing. They strive to be relevant, truthful, clear, and informative (Grice, 1975). Their messages are long enough to make the point (but not overly long), relate to previous messages, and pro- voke further thought or discussion. Skilled communicators also adapt their language to their audience, monitor for comprehension, and use good judg- ment in pacing and timing.

Nonverbal Communication

Most of us began life with a cry, a vocal but nonverbal communication. Throughout our lives, we continue to use nonverbal communication to com- plement our verbal messages or, in some cases, complicate them, as in the case of sarcasm. Physical aspects of nonverbal communication include body pos- ture and proximity, gesture, touch, eye gaze behavior, and facial expression. Vocal aspects of nonverbal communication include voice quality, pitch, rate, volume, and prosody (rhythm, intonation, and stress). Other paralinguistic features include hesitations *(uh, um)*, yawns, sighs, laughs, cries, and pauses. Few people are aware of all of these features of nonverbal communication and even fewer receive formal training in interpreting and controlling these sig- nals. All of us can build on our tacit understanding of nonverbal communica- tion by careful observation and reflection.

EXERCISE 4.2

The Center for Nonverbal Studies maintains an online Nonverbal Diction- ary (Givens, 2015) with hundreds of entries.[1] Use the dictionary to answer the following questions:

What might hand-behind-head signify? How would putting both hands behind the head be different?

_____

_____

_____

How are head-tilt-back and head-tilt-side different? Are these signals the same across cultures?

_____

_____

_____

Knapp and Hall (2002, pp. 253–260) reviewed the many ways that we use nonverbal behavior to regulate social interactions. Conversational involvement may be signaled by postural congruence, mimicry of facial expression, and meshing of changes in movement. Listener back-channel vocalizations *(mmm-hmm, I see, yeah)*, head nods, and movements of the hands and feet are often synchronized with the speaker's rhythms. Conversational partners may match loudness, precision of articulation, speech rate, and duration of pauses and utterances. Initiating and turn-taking in conversations are also regulated by nonverbal and paralinguistic cues, including changes in eye contact, eyebrow flashes, postural adjustments, gestures, head nods, pauses, audible breaths, and conversational trailers such as *you know . . ., so . . ., ah . . .* (Knapp & Hall, 2002, p. 18).

How people interact with the physical environment is another aspect of nonverbal communication. Research on small-group ecology provides useful insights on how seating behavior and spatial arrangements communicate expectations for working collaboratively (Knapp & Hall, 2002, pp. 161–164):

- Leadership and dominance are associated with seats at the end of a rectangular table.
- Task-oriented leaders are attracted to seats at the end of the table, while leaders oriented toward group maintenance opt for visually central seats.
- Cooperation is associated with side-by-side seating, while competition is associated with opposite seating.

Clearly, the environment can have significant effects on social interactions; for example, a lecture theater with fixed seating discourages peer interaction. Lighting, noise, temperature, seating comfort, and floor plans are other environmental factors that affect communication patterns and styles (Knapp & Hall, 2002, pp. 117–134).

Paralinguistic cues can provide strong signals of confidence and authority. Inspection of legal court transcripts has led to constructs of powerful and powerless speech styles that have been verified in other settings (Hosman, 1989). Specifically, perceptions of a speaker's authoritativeness are negatively affected by hesitations *(um, er)* and hedges *(sort of, kind of)*. Intensifiers *(very, definitely, really)* are perceived as powerful, but only in the absence of hesitations or hedges. Hosman pointed out that there may be an upper limit to how these cues signal authority: "Speakers who are too sure of their ideas, do not hedge, and do intensify may be perceived as dogmatic, unsociable, and dishonest" (1989, p. 402).

Different social groups vary in how they use nonverbal communication. Ethnicity, gender, and socio-economic factors all contribute to social identity and communication norms. When people are unaware of different norms for nonverbal signals, stereotypes may be triggered and misunderstandings may occur. For example, Shokeir (2008) found that adult women of all ages used uptalk — a rising contour at the end of declarative sentences — more than men, and that men were more likely than women to interpret uptalk as signaling uncertainty and continuation. In another example, non-Aboriginal physicians serving some Aboriginal communities in Canada recounted how they learned to communicate respect to their patients and co-workers by abiding long pauses and avoiding eye contact (Kelly & Brown, 2002). More generally, years of research from different countries supports the observation that people who speak with the standard accent of the dominant group are given higher status ratings than those who speak with foreign or regional non-standard accents (Fuertes, Potere, & Ramirez, 2002). Note that context mediates such evaluations: speakers with non-standard accents are rated less negatively in informal settings.

You get people in the group who do not want to share their opinions.

Overall, research on nonverbal communication highlights the importance of context for using and interpreting nonverbal signals. Since part of the context is the actual content of the message, let us turn to consider effective ways to communicate that content.

Spoken Language

When we speak, we exploit the tremendous power of human language. Language transcends time, place, and person — it allows us to talk of future possibilities, to relate past experiences, to express who we are. With the power of language comes responsibility, especially in healthcare: to use that power in the service of efficacious and ethical patient- and family-centered care. In this section, we consider how we may unwittingly jeopardize our pursuit of these goals by ignoring important characteristics of words and sentences, such as ambiguity, overgeneralization, and polarization.

Words, the basic elements of spoken language, are arbitrary signals used to communicate thoughts and feelings. In addition to their primary meaning or dictionary definition, known as denotations, words also have connotations — secondary associations that often carry emotional significance. For this reason, words may represent different things to different people or in different contexts. Many words are inherently ambiguous: the word *run* has dozens of distinct definitions, and homophones (two different words that sound the same, such as *sole* and *soul*) are ambiguous out of context when spoken. Skilled communicators are mindful of connotative meaning and potential ambiguity when they choose which words to use.

EXERCISE 4.3

Consider the use of the word *complaint* in healthcare. Many health professionals learn to identify and document a patient's chief complaint. This can lead to the use of the word *complaint* in conversation, such as saying, "The mother complains that the child is constipated."

How might the connotations of the word complaint *affect communication with patients, families, and other health professionals?*

_____

_____

_____

Think of some alternatives to the word complaint *for this kind of communication.*

_____

_____

_____

What other words commonly used in healthcare have undesirable connotations?

_____

_____

_____

Misunderstanding of words is more likely when intelligibility is reduced, when the context is unclear, or when people speak different regional dialects of a language. When meaning is unclear, listeners may fill in the missing information with content from their own experience (Ludden, 2002), such as the student who sat through a lecture hearing *hydrogen bombs* instead of *hydrogen bonds*. Some misunderstandings are trivial, but a misheard medication order, for example, may be serious. To prevent misunderstanding, effective communicators speak clearly, enhance intelligibility by reducing noise or using a microphone, establish the context, and use vocabulary that is most familiar to the listener. When safety is important, the message should be confirmed in writing or by using closed loop communication (described in the last section of this chapter).

EXERCISE 4.4

The website of the World Health Organization (2007) has resources for patient safety, including an article about the risks associated with look-alike, sound-alike medication names. Study this article[2] and then answer the following questions:

How many trademarked and non-proprietary medication names have been reported in the United States?

_____

_____

_____

What strategies does the World Health Organization suggest to manage risks associated with look-alike, sound-alike medications?

_____

_____

_____

How can patients and caregivers help reduce these risks?

_____

_____

_____

Jargon and acronyms convey information quickly and contribute to a sense of group identity when there is a shared understanding of their meaning. Problems arise when there isn't a shared understanding, especially when members of a group don't realize that a term or acronym means different things to different people. In addition, use of jargon and acronyms may alienate newcomers; time must be taken to explain jargon and newcomers are justified in asking for explanations. When undefined acronyms are used in a flyer or in an email subject line to advertise an event, opportunities to engage new people may be missed. For these reasons, good communicators use jargon sparingly and judiciously.

Words are assembled into phrases, sentences, and longer chunks of discourse following the rules and conventions of a language. Poor grammar and organization in speech can obscure the message, distract the listener, and create a negative impression of the speaker. Even when the grammar and structure of a passage are clear, verbal communication can lead to various problems (Klinzing & Klinzing, 1985, pp. 69–74):

- **Fact/Inference confusions:** Factual statements (e.g., *The patient did not respond when I greeted her this morning*) are verifiable observations about the past or present, while inferential statements (e.g., *She has a bad attitude*) have varying degrees of probability. Speakers may not give clear cues to differentiate statements of fact and inference; indeed, the tone of an inferential statement may give it the weight of fact.
- **Overgeneralization:** Superordinate nouns (e.g., *nurses, foreigners, scholars, addicts*) and non-specific verbs (e.g., *are, go, do, use*) emphasize similarities rather than differences and thus contribute to stereotypes. Modifiers such as *all, every, always,* and *never* are strong markers for overgeneralization. These features of language also lead us to think of individuals or situations as static rather than changing over time.
- **Polarization:** Polar terms (e.g., *short/tall, success/failure, right/wrong, cooperative/uncooperative, good/bad*) promote thinking in terms of dichotomies or false choices. Such black-and-white language often misrepresents reality and prevents communicators from appreciating complexities.

Competent communicators minimize these problems by considering carefully what they want to say and how they want to say it. They introduce inferential statements with phrases such as *I believe that . . ., I wonder if . . .,* or *It seems that . . .* They avoid words that overgeneralize or polarize and use qualifiers (e.g., *some, many, few, sometimes, often, usually*) when needed.

Skilled communicators in small groups monitor listeners' comprehension by observing nonverbal cues and interacting with listeners to ask questions or check assumptions. They also adapt their speaking style to suit the listener, something even young children have been observed to do. Nevertheless, Keysar and Henly (2002) found that speakers overestimated how well they were understood when they attempted to convey a specific meaning while saying an ambiguous sentence (see also Fay, Page, & Serfaty, 2010). These researchers also found that bystanders who overheard the speaker assessed the speaker's communicative effectiveness accurately. These findings reinforce the principle that effective communication requires active participation by all group members: speakers, listeners, and bystanders.

Active Listening

Conversation is collaborative, not a competitive sport where the first one to take a breath is considered the listener (Miller, 1965, p. 83). Listeners share responsibility with speakers for ensuring that a message is complete, accurate, and understandable. To carry out this responsibility, active listeners do the following:

- Reconcile verbal information with nonverbal signals
- Reflect feelings
- Ask questions for clarification
- Paraphrase the speaker's message

By attending to both the rational and emotional content of a message, listeners are more likely to understand the speaker's intent as well as the speaker's values and potential for being in conflict.

Pico Iyer recently wrote, "In an age of distraction, nothing can feel more luxurious than paying attention" (2014, p. 65). The first step of paying attention is to stop talking and to start listening and observing. While this step is obvious, it is not always easy to achieve for the following reasons (Klinzing & Klinzing, 1985, pp. 45–62):

- Our minds work faster than the pace of spoken words, potentially leading to a loss of focus.
- We listen through our own filters and mental set, leading us to alter the intended meaning.
- We often start to think about the content and even plan our response before we have listened to the entire message.

In other words, if we don't work at listening, all we hear is ourselves.

As the term implies, active listening is not passive and requires effort. The listener must become "a collaborator in the communication process" (McKay, Davis, & Fanning, 2009, p. 17). To this end, listeners may intentionally exhibit nonverbal behavior to show that they are listening, such as sitting down, leaning forward, facing the speaker, making eye contact, and using open posture (Weger, Castle, & Emmett, 2010). By using these nonverbal signals, listeners convey their openness to the speaker and the speaker's message.

Some people are not willing to see others' opinions — they're not open-minded.

External events may interfere with listening. People, pagers, or telephone calls may interrupt the interaction. Noise in the environment — such as voices in a hallway, clattering carts, or machinery noise — can significantly affect the intelligibility of speech and the mental effort required for listening (Rashid & Zimring, 2008; Sarampalis, Kalluri, Edwards, & Hafter, 2009). To reduce the effect of these distractions, listeners may choose to close a door, move closer to the speaker, and turn off sounds from electronic devices. These actions all demonstrate the respect of the listener for the speaker and improve the likelihood of effective communication.

EXERCISE 4.5

Make a copy of the active listening checklist in Appendix C and use it to guide your observations of a communication interaction, with permission from the people you are observing.

What signals tell you that someone is actively listening?

_____

_____

_____

What effect does multitasking, such as using electronic devices, have on these signals?

_____

_____

_____

What ground rules might a group want to establish about using electronic devices during meetings?

_____

_____

_____

Internal events may also interfere with listening. Listeners may find themselves faking or losing attention if they are stressed or preoccupied. They may be distracted by particular words or phrases or by the speaker's appearance, voice quality, or speech patterns. To counteract these internal distractions, listeners need to engage in self-monitoring and take corrective actions, which can be as simple as sitting up straighter or as complex as the following:

- Listeners who notice that they are stressed or preoccupied should take steps to manage their stress. In addition, they may choose to share information about how they are feeling with their colleagues, ask to resume the discussion at another time, or shelve their preoccupation in order regain focus on the work of active listening.

- Listeners who notice that they are distracted or faking attention can utilize the speed-of-thought advantage by devoting mental effort toward reconciling the speaker's verbal and nonverbal messages and considering the speaker's context, values, and emotions.
- Listeners who notice that certain words or phrases trigger emotional responses or tangential thoughts may choose to engage in emotion regulation, ask questions for clarification, or make a mental note of their reactions for later reflection.
- Listeners who notice that they are indulging in stereotyping can resolve to suspend judgment and be tolerant, look for counterexamples to their stereotypes, and/or remind themselves of the value of diverse points of view in collaboration.

By taking steps to reduce external and internal distractions, listeners increase their ability to grasp the essence of what is being said.

In short, active listening requires considerable internal activity coupled with external signals of calm receptivity — like a duck moving upriver that appears serene but whose feet are paddling furiously underwater. Fortunately, investing energy in active listening provides ample rewards. Active listening contributes to quality healthcare as well as to satisfying and positive interprofessional relationships (Gilbert, Ussher, Perz, Hobbs, & Kirsten, 2010; Warshawsky, Havens, & Knafl, 2012). When listeners convey empathy and respect, speakers are empowered to state more clearly their own needs and concerns. Active listening leads to learning — the listener will be changed in some way by the message received (Ludden, 2002).

Asynchronous Communication

Face-to-face and telephone communications happen synchronously, allowing participants to integrate verbal and nonverbal signals and build on each other's contributions. Communication with a time lag, such as voice mail, email, a chart note, or a letter, is asynchronous. The degree of time lag varies across a large spectrum depending on what communication system is used and how frequently participants engage with that system. The degree of interactivity also varies across systems. While voice mail, sound recordings, or video recordings may be used, most asynchronous communication in healthcare is written.

Writing

Effective healthcare depends on written language: health professionals write reports, chart notes, letters, minutes, memos, agendas, and proposals. Clinical documentation is so important in healthcare that it is often said that "if it isn't documented, it didn't happen" (Boone, 2011, chap. 2). In addition to traditional forms of documentation, computer-mediated communication systems such as email, instant messaging, and texting have become increasingly important to many work groups.

Writing has some advantages over speaking. For example, written work can be edited to increase its accuracy, brevity, clarity, and relevance. Written communication may be financially efficient: it serves those unable to meet in the same time or space and may take less time than a phone call or face-to-face meeting. Written communication can potentially reach all intended recipients and can be stored for future reference.

I don't think we need to meet as a group. Email works just as well.

Written communication has the disadvantage of being less immediate and more easily ignored or forgotten than face-to-face interactions. Because of time lags, written communication may arrive too late to be useful to the collaborative process, though current technologies increase the speed of exchange. Even so, Gottesdiener (2002) suggests that over-reliance on technology can actually distance group members and create opportunities for miscommunication. Indeed, some communication technologies are so convenient and accessible that they increase the risk that a message may be sent in anger or frustration. Effective communicators recognize these limitations, find the right balance of written and spoken communication, and create shared ground rules for how they communicate.

VIGNETTE 4.1

During an evening shift, a team of physicians proposes to discharge a patient from a pediatric acute care unit in the morning if he continues to do well overnight. They write a brief note in the chart summarizing this plan. At morning rounds, the medical team gives an overview of the patient's hospital course and writes the discharge order.

Later in the afternoon, the patient's therapists arrive on the unit and are exasperated when the nurse tells them that the patient has gone home.

What are the positive and negative consequences of the way written communication was used in this situation?

What are the potential reasons for the breakdown in communication?

How might these individuals and/or this organization improve interprofessional communication?

When composing written messages, it is important to remember that they may be distributed beyond the intended audience. While oral communication can certainly be relayed to others after the original exchange, people generally reserve judgment about second-hand, word-of-mouth information, as illustrated by the connotations of the following synonyms: hearsay, rumor, grapevine, scuttlebutt, or gossip. In contrast, written communication may be circulated in its original form, appearing more authentic to readers who may not have the context or background to understand the original intent. Many organizations now stress that computer-mediated messaging is not private and encourage employees to consider all such communications to be equivalent to public announcements. In other words, compose your email message as if it will be read aloud in the cafeteria — if you wouldn't want that, don't write it.

Reading

One major limitation of written communication is the absence of the nonverbal channel. As the phrase *reading between the lines* suggests, actively processing written communication requires making inferences about the intended meaning and tone. Without nonverbal cues, the reader may misinterpret the tone of the message and the writer may not know how the message was received.

Writers of formal letters and official memos often introduce their main message with a statement of feeling: *We regret to inform you . . ., I am pleased to announce . . ., Thank you for your referral . . .* Such introductory statements prepare the reader for the content and provide some context about the intended tone and meaning. Writers using informal communication methods such as email, texting, or messaging may not take as much time or care to compose their message. While emoticons may help clarify the tone in informal communication, their effect may not always be beneficial. For example, a research study found that negative emoticons in task-oriented messages intensified the message and worsened the recipient's negative emotion (Luor, Wu, Lu, & Tao, 2010). Even informal messages need to be crafted carefully to be informative, constructive, and transparent.

The internal and external factors that affect reading are similar to those affecting listening. Interruptions, poor script legibility, and low light levels can reduce reading accuracy. Like listeners, readers may find themselves functioning in an automatic way, or being distracted by words, phrases, grammar, or spelling. Readers, however, have the advantage of being able to reread passages and process the written word at their own pace. To engage with text more actively, readers may choose to underline words or phrases, make annotations, or take notes.

For long documents, proficient readers apply metacognitive skills: thinking about thinking, monitoring, and self-regulating. The SQ3R is a popular method for teaching these metacognitive skills and improving reading proficiency in post-secondary students. In this method, readers survey (S) or skim the text quickly for the main points and structure, ask questions (Q) and make predictions about the author's intent, read (R1) in a focused way, making notes if desired, recite (R2) and reflect, checking for comprehension, and finally review (R3) and summarize in their own words. Active reading, like active listening, allows readers to improve their comprehension and retention (Artis, 2008; Lei, Rhinehart, Howard, & Cho, 2010).

Because written words endure and because they lack the give and take of spoken conversation with its nonverbal cues, written words may have even more power than spoken words. Readers who find themselves emotionally affected or troubled by what they read could do the following:

- Reread from the writer's perspective: What did the writer most likely intend?
- Consider any seemingly irrelevant or misleading statements, exaggerations, generalizations, or polarizations: Is there a constructive or valuable underlying message?
- Contact the writer and engage in conversation instead of replying by email or with another memo: What goals do you have for this conversation? For the relationship?

More information about having difficult conversations appears later in this chapter. First, let us consider the value of informal communication in building collaborative relationships.

Informal Communication

Informal communication includes unstructured conversations that occur in a hallway, a coffee room, over lunch, or at social events. Such conversations help build work relationships and social networks. Although some may view informal communication in an organizational context as frivolous, research shows that more knowledge is shared through informal communication than through formal communication (Ipe, 2003). Within the constraints of maintaining appropriate boundaries and work relationships, social time is valuable for sharing ideas as well as for team building and maintenance.

In his book *Social Physics*, Pentland (2014) explains how new research methods using enormous data sets have provided insights into the importance of informal communication. In one study, the manager of a call center for a major bank wanted to understand why there was wide variation in productivity among seemingly identical work teams (Waber, Olguin Olguin, Kim, & Pentland, 2010). The researchers asked members of four teams at this call center to wear electronic badges

Time gets wasted getting to know everyone.

that recorded, among other things, who spoke to whom, when, how much, tone of voice, and body language. Analysis of six weeks of detailed behavioral data showed that the best predictors of productivity were team members' energy and engagement outside of formal meetings. The researchers then recommended that all members of a team take a coffee break at the same time (rather than having staggered breaks) to provide them with some group time away from their workstations. Counterintuitively, this intervention led to significant increases in productivity, engagement, and employee satisfaction, especially among the least productive teams. These researchers concluded that "strong social groups are beneficial to productivity and can be supported without extensive management interventions" (Waber et al., 2010, p. 15).

Some groups routinely incorporate informal communication at the beginning of a meeting. For example, group members may make a brief personal statement about how they are feeling, significant events in their lives, or what they hope to accomplish in the meeting. Groups who implement this kind of check-in at the beginning of a meeting may wish to experiment with different ground rules, such as having an option to pass (remain silent), permitting or disallowing interactive conversations, and setting time limits. By finding out about each other's current moods, preoccupations, or goals, group members strengthen their relationships and develop deeper appreciation of their colleagues as multidimensional individuals. They are also less likely to misinterpret each other's verbal and nonverbal signals and more likely to speak up when needed.

Self-Awareness

Many practitioners and educators in healthcare point to the importance of self-awareness and self-reflection for professional development. Clark (1997), for example, discussed how conflicts in collaborative care for the elderly are better couched as conflicts of values than conflicts of roles and called for interprofessional education to help students to identify their values as part of their professional identity. Medical educators and learners have been urged to "consciously attend to their relationships and

---

VIGNETTE 4.2

Four members of a research team in different cities meet regularly online to work on a grant proposal. They are unsatisfied with their progress and feel they lack focus during their meetings. By mutual agreement, they resolve to start each session with a check-in. Each person has two minutes to talk about any personal thoughts and experiences he or she wishes to share. All others remain silent for the full two minutes. One person keeps track of the time.

How might this check-in process improve task-focused communication?

Why might a group that meets online choose to use a structured check-in process such as this?

What role would a similar process have in a face-to-face meeting?

work on self-awareness and mindfulness" rather than deferring insights about the human side of medicine to a mid-career epiphany (Dobie, 2007, p. 422). Ünal (2012) described how undergraduate nurses developed self-awareness as they learned to apply communication and assertiveness skills. Communicators who are aware of their own attitudes, beliefs, values, and goals are able to send clear messages and attend well to others' messages (Beebe, Beebe, Redmond, & Geerinck, 2004).

Attitudes and Beliefs

In chapter 2, we presented information about the Attitudes toward Health Care Teams Scale (Heinemann et al., 1999). Using this tool helps individuals examine their own attitudes and beliefs about collaborating with other health professionals. It can also help group members explore their similarities and differences as they build a shared mental model of their goals and processes. While listening to others may change our attitudes and beliefs as we gain new understandings, participatory decision making does not require that all group members have identical attitudes and beliefs — we can agree to disagree.

Stereotypes are beliefs about others that help us fill in information based on previously established biases. The social pragmatic utility of stereotypes is to improve efficiency as we recognize and respond to situations that we have previously encountered (Beebe et al., 2004). As the diversity of a group increases, so do opportunities for stereotypes to influence communication both overtly and insidiously. As explained in chapter 2, diversity of personal characteristics (gender, age, culture, ethnicity, and education) and occupational characteristics (occupation, rank, income, and status) can either enhance or undermine group effectiveness.

We don't know enough about what each other does.

Stereotypes about healthcare professions may initially inform group members about the roles and responsibilities of other members and how they are likely to function in a group (Carpenter, 1995; Cragan & Wright, 1999). Whether positive or negative, such stereotypes are often strengthened by experience, even in early stages of professional education (Mandy, Milton, & Mandy, 2004). We tend to seek and remember information that reinforces our beliefs, a phenomenon known as confirmation bias (Fiske, 1998).

Research has demonstrated that it is possible, though difficult, to become aware of one's biases and to challenge them (Fiske, 1998). Looking for counter-examples to previously established biases helps undo the universal tendency to overgeneralize and improves communication competence (Beebe et al., 2004). In this way, listeners with insight about their own stereotypes of others can strive to reduce their filtering effect. Similarly, speakers who are aware of what

VIGNETTE 4.3

A psychologist completes a psycho-educational assessment of a teen with attention-deficit hyperactivity disorder at the request of a physician. The psychologist arranges a case conference with the teen, the parent, the school personnel, and the referring physician for both information sharing and determining resource needs.

When the physician arrives at the meeting, she finds that a chair is reserved for her at the head of the table. When the meeting starts, the physician is surprised when all the participants look to her to run the meeting.

What assumptions led to this situation?

What problems could arise due to these assumptions?

How might stereotyping by and of health professionals contribute to mistaken assumptions?

stereotypes they may engender can strategically construct messages designed to expand how others see them. In other words, health professionals can make it easier for others to dispel stereotypes by taking initiative to express their own values and to explain how they see their role and responsibilities.

Values and Goals

Values drive our behavior: we act to get things done and also to confirm our self-worth by acting in ways congruent with our values. Within any working group, people differ in how they prioritize values such as achievement, altruism, rationality, and flexibility. Individuals feel more satisfied with their collaborative work when their most deeply held values are affirmed (Porter, 1996). Recognizing our own core values while acknowledging that others have different priorities guides our communication behavior and helps us understand the behavior of our colleagues, especially during times of conflict. Furthermore, communicators are more likely to engage listeners when they adapt their communication style and focus to listeners' values and orientation (see Table 4.1).

TABLE 4.1 MATCHING COMMUNICATION STYLE AND FOCUS TO LISTENER ORIENTATION AND VALUES

ORIENTATION	PREDOMINANT VALUES	STYLE	FOCUS
Action	Achievement Productivity	Brief Practical	Results and challenges
Process	Rationality Accuracy	Precise Logical	Pros and cons to alternative options
Relationship	Altruism Harmony	Informal Empathetic	Opinions and endorsements of others
Conceptual	Creativity Flexibility	Provocative Expansive	Ideas and possibilities

Source: Adapted from R. Youker (2013). Using the communications styles instrument for teambuilding. *PM World Journal, 2*(7).

EXERCISE 4.6

In 2013, Robert Youker made available online his Communication Styles Inventory via the *PM World Journal*, a global resource for sharing knowledge in program and project management. Download this inventory[3] and complete it for yourself:

What is your predominant communication style?

_____

_____

_____

What values does this style reflect?

_____

_____

_____

What strengths do you offer to collaborative work?

_____

_____

_____

How might you adapt your style to work with someone with different strengths?

_____

_____

_____

We carry our values with us from one situation to another, but our goals are usually situation-specific. Being aware of one's real purpose, as well as one's values, wants, and needs, is the only way to prepare to give a complete and forthright message (McKay, Davis, & Fanning, 2009, p. 52). In their book *Crucial Conversations*, Patterson, Grenny, McMillan, and Switzler (2012) noted that when opinions vary and stakes are high, skilled communicators stay focused on their goals.

Hidden agendas are incompatible with communication for collaboration. When group members deliberately use a group for a hidden purpose, they violate the principles of honesty and mutual understanding, both of which are fundamental to shared leadership and participatory decision making. More commonly, group members may not be fully aware of their own motives. Patterson et al. found that skilled communicators are honest with themselves about the story or rationale behind the feelings that they experience — they consider what their behavior reveals about what their motives are and then ask themselves, "What do I want for myself? For others? For the relationship?" (2012, p. 48). Equipped with this self-awareness, skilled communicators take action to increase feelings of safety and respect during difficult conversations to keep the dialogue moving forward.

Focusing on goals promotes collaboration and helps communicators prevent or manage conflict, especially when there is a power differential (e.g., among health professionals or between health professionals and patients/ family members). McNaughton and Vostal (2010) presented "LAFF don't CRY" as a framework for training teachers to stay focused on goals when dealing with parents' concerns. Instead of responding to a complaint or concern by *criticizing* or blaming people who aren't present (C), *reacting* hastily and promising something that can't be delivered (R), or *yakking* on about personal experiences to shift attention away from the problem at hand (Y), professionals learn to do the following:

- **Listen, empathize, and communicate respect (L):** Use nonverbal cues to signal openness and empathy; restate and/or validate the speaker's concern; thank the speaker for bringing the issue forward.
- ***Ask* questions and ask permission to take notes (A):** Gather information to learn more about the speaker's perspective and relevant details; take notes to focus on the problem and document the conversation.
- ***Focus* on the issues (F):** Review and check for accuracy.
- ***Find* a first step (F):** Work out an immediate goal, which can be as simple as "Let's meet again tomorrow."

These skills for active listening and goal-focused communication move a conversation full circle — from complaint to an initial step toward resolution. Not every conversation will lead immediately to a full resolution; in fact, participants often benefit from additional time to reflect and gather more information toward finding a solution that works for everyone. Research supports the validity and utility of this system: parents from diverse linguistic and cultural backgrounds rated student teachers to be better communicators once those students had learned how to follow the LAFF framework (McNaughton, Hamlin, McCarthy, Head-Reeves, & Schreiner, 2008).

To summarize, self-awareness facilitates good communication when speakers and listeners have insight into their own attitudes, beliefs, values, and goals. Health professionals who maintain a high level of self-awareness are more open to new information and better able to express themselves productively, particularly in difficult or crucial conversations. Self-awareness allows collaborators to find mutually acceptable solutions to problems without sacrificing deeply held values and beliefs.

Communication Tools

Health professionals can draw from a wide array of communication strategies and tools to support effective interprofessional collaboration and manage conflict. We have already described adapting to others' values and communication style, check-ins, alternatives to open discussion (listed in the conflict management section of chapter 3) and goal-focused frameworks (e.g., LAFF). In this section, we briefly present some other tools: structured reflection, three frameworks for establishing expectations for communication in interprofessional collaboration (SCRIPT, SBAR, and CORBS), and closed loop communication.

Structured Reflection

Having seen how important self-awareness is to effective communication, we can understand why reflection is becoming an increasingly popular approach to improving healthcare practice and education. Reflection can be done by structured classroom exercises, by self-study (e.g., checklists, journals), or by peer support groups (McLeod, 2003). In the domain of communication, some topics for reflection may include the following:

- What message do I need or want to send? Is the message intended to achieve a common goal or a personal goal (e.g., preservation of self-worth)?
- Am I free to convey the content of my message or am I restricted in some way, such as by confidentiality? Is the timing acceptable?
- How do my attitudes and beliefs affect what I say and how I listen? How do others' attitudes and beliefs affect how they perceive me and how I perceive them?
- When conflicts have arisen, what part of the message relates to the common goal and what relates to group maintenance?
- How will this message be received by different people? How may it threaten others? Are there other solutions?

While maintaining self-awareness during conversations can be difficult, structured reflection before and after conversations can help untangle the complex weaving of meaning, attitudes, beliefs, goals, and values.

SCRIPT

Structuring Communication Relationships for Interprofessional Teamwork (SCRIPT) is a program for encouraging reciprocal communication patterns among health professionals outside of structured meetings (Zwarenstein et al., 2007). In this program, health professionals and trainees who have face-to-face patient-related interactions with others from different professional backgrounds learn to follow these steps:

I don't think people appreciate and acknowledge what people in my profession can do.

- **Name:** Introduce yourself by name and title.
- **Role:** State your professional role with the team, unit, or department and describe your role in relation to the patient under discussion.
- **Issue:** Share with others your profession-specific problem or plan as it relates to the patient under discussion.
- **Feedback:** Elicit interaction-specific feedback from other participants by asking questions such as *Do you have any concerns?* or *Is there something else I should consider?*

By following these steps, health professionals in knotworks or template teams reduce anonymity, clarify roles, identify problems and goals, and become more engaged in productive collaboration. While the framework is simple and straightforward, research has shown that uptake of this framework may be impeded in some settings by professional resistance, power differentials, or by fast-paced environments that offer few opportunities or incentives to enhance interprofessional relationships (Rice et al., 2010; Zwarenstein, Rice, Gotlib-Conn, Kenaszchuk, & Reeves, 2013). Such research illustrates that improving communication competence among practicing health professionals requires attention to all levels of operation: interpersonal, organizational, and systemic.

SBAR

Situation, Background, Assessment, and Recommendation (SBAR) is a template for what to include and what response to expect in a communication exchange between health professionals collaborating in a clinical situation (Haig, Sutton, & Whittington, 2006; Institute for Healthcare Improvement, n.d.). The template follows this format:

- **Situation:** Describe the situation; state your name, position, work setting, topic, time needed to discuss (if not now, when?).
- **Background:** Provide background information about the specific problem; for example, patient name, diagnosis, admission date, scheduled

discharge date, treatment plan, names of specialists, planned procedures, patient/family/staff request.

- **Assessment:** Provide your assessment of the key underlying problem/concern, key changes since last assessment (patient vital signs/characteristics, patient participation/activity/function, environmental).

- **Recommendation:** Provide your recommendation, summarize, and confirm: *Based on this assessment, I recommend that . . . Are you okay with this plan? To be clear, we agreed to . . .*

In addition to supporting efficient communication, SBAR empowers those who need to send a message to someone with more power or status, and makes it clear to the receiver that an action is required. SBAR has been demonstrated to improve communication skills and patient safety (De Meester, Verspuy, Monsieurs, & Van Bogaert, 2013; Marshall, Harrison, & Flanagan, 2009).

CORBS

Clear, Owned, Regular, Balanced, and Specific (CORBS) is a set of guidelines for giving feedback effectively (Hawkins & Shohet, 2006, pp. 133–135). Providing feedback to others is a core competency for training situations (teaching and supervision) as well as for professional practice (leadership and teamwork). While giving and receiving feedback can be anxiety provoking, following these guidelines increases the likelihood that feedback will be productive and will lead to learning and behavior change:

- **Clear:** Give clear and concise information to reduce anxiety and be understood.
- **Owned:** Recognize that your feedback says as much about you as it does about the recipient of the feedback. Describe your own perceptions using phrases such as *I find . . .* or *When you . . . I felt . . .* rather than *You are . . .*
- **Regular:** Offer feedback regularly; that is, immediately or as close to the event as possible, rather than saving it up for another time.
- **Balanced:** Balance negative feedback with positive feedback over time.
- **Specific:** Comment on observable behavior and behavior that can be modified.

CORBS has research support for its utility and efficacy in training situations (Motley, Reese, & Campos, 2014). CORBS can also be applied to interprofessional practice when colleagues provide feedback to each other as part of the process of mutual support in teamwork (Alonso & Dunleavy, 2013).

Closed Loop Communication

This communication technique ensures that the message was received and interpreted correctly. To close the loop, the receiver makes eye contact (if possible) and repeats the message back to the sender who either confirms that the message was received correctly or identifies and corrects the error. Closed loop communication is particularly useful when the risks associated with miscommunication are high, such as during an emergency or a highly coordinated or technical activity, all of which are common in healthcare (Burke, Salas, Wilson-Donnelly, & Priest, 2004; Salas, Wilson, Murphy, King, & Salisbury, 2008). Closed loop communication is commonly used when medication orders are given orally (e.g., by telephone) under urgent circumstances; that is, when a patient's safety and care would be compromised if time were taken to send a written message or when it is not possible to send a written message. In situations with lower risk, closed loop communication can be used when discussions get heated or when some group members get left behind to slow down the pace of communication and increase mutual understanding.

EXERCISE 4.7

Draft a short proposal to advocate for communication training for your working group.

What kind of training would you suggest? For what purpose?

_____

_____

_____

What barriers or misconceptions must be addressed to secure the interest and engagement of members of your working group in this training?

_____

_____

_____

What organizational supports would be needed to foster implementation of this training in daily practice?

_____

_____

_____

Applying the Framework

In this chapter, you learned about the values, skills, and knowledge underlying effective communication for interprofessional collaboration. Communication competence is needed at all levels of interaction — interpersonal, organizational, and systemic (see Table 4.2). Vignette 4.1 illustrates how communication competence is needed at the organizational level to provide timely information to other members of a team or knotwork. Vignette 4.2 illustrates how communication competence is needed at the interpersonal level to support mutual understanding. Vignette 4.3 illustrates how communication competence is needed at the systemic level to be aware of stereotypes and to check assumptions.

TABLE 4.2 FRAMEWORK FOR COMMUNICATION

	INTERPERSONAL	ORGANIZATIONAL	SYSTEMIC
Communication	Mutual understanding	Timeliness	Stereotypes

EXERCISE 4.8

Reflect on your own experiences of communication for collaboration and answer the following questions:

What keywords can you add to the cells in the framework in Table 4.2 that pertain to each of your stories?

_____

_____

_____

How might this framework inform your analysis of these stories?

_____

_____

_____

Like teamwork and leadership, communication is learned behavior. Moreover, communication competencies are critical to interprofessional collaboration — without effective communication, teamwork and leadership competencies may lie dormant. By understanding the challenges of communication in small groups, sending clear verbal and nonverbal signals, listening actively, and developing insight into your own values, goals, and filters, you can engage in productive interactions like those described at the beginning of this chapter. Your team discussion is easy and worry-free, you have confidence that the messages sent are the ones intended to be sent, and those listening receive those messages in the way they were intended.

Mastering competencies for teamwork, leadership, and communication is a lifelong enterprise, with many twists and turns along the path. As you set out to collaborate with others, it is important to know where you are heading. In the next and final chapter, we provide a road map to guide you on your way.

NOTES

1 www.center-for-nonverbal-studies.org/6101.html

2 http://www.who.int/patientsafety/solutions/patientsafety/PS-Solution1.pdf

3 www.pmworldlibrary.net/

5

Weaving the Fabric of Collaboration

Imagine collaborating with others toward a common goal, following a mutually agreed upon process, resolving differences, evaluating outcomes, and celebrating successes...

AFTER READING THIS CHAPTER, YOU WILL BE ABLE TO DO THE FOLLOWING:

- Describe how to build a *shared mental model* for collaboration by mapping out a group's goals and process, clarifying professional roles and boundaries, and contributing knowledge of resources
- Demonstrate *engagement* and *integrity* in collaboration
- Select a suitable tool or process for *assessment* and *evaluation* of individual competencies and of groups, teams, or systems
- *Apply the framework* for reflection and problem solving

Equipped with competencies in teamwork, leadership, and communication, health professionals are ready to take action and put theory into practice. As a first step, group members need a shared mental model — a blueprint for their work together. That mental model includes knowledge of the group's goals and tasks as well as how the group works together and makes decisions. Group members need to have a clear understanding of their own roles and boundaries and of others' roles and boundaries, including expectations for confidentiality. Groups need adequate resources to accomplish their goals, awareness of available resources, and ways to remedy resource deficiencies. When group members are fully engaged in collaborative work and demonstrate integrity in their relationships, they can resolve problems and move forward with confidence. Responsible groups evaluate their work by using specific tools or building evaluation into their standard procedures.

Shared Mental Model

To understand what drives successful collaboration, researchers use the construct of team cognition (Salas & Fiore, 2004). Team cognition refers to the

collective cognitive, behavioral, and attitudinal activity of members of a collaborative group. By applying the ideas and methods of cognitive psychology
to those of organizational and social psychology, the team cognition movement has started to develop "theoretically driven and empirically based guidelines for designing, managing, and developing teams" (Salas & Fiore, 2004,
p. 4). One emerging guideline is that groups benefit from building a shared
mental model of the group's process and its product (Fiore & Schooler, 2004).

Goals and Process

It seems obvious that collaboration must start with a shared understanding
of the goals or desired outcomes of the group, but omitting this step is common. While group members may be impatient to start on their "real" work, it
is essential to take time to make sure everyone develops a shared understanding of what that real work is. That shared understanding includes a vision
of the overarching goal, what steps are needed toward that goal, and what
tasks need to be done. As well, group members need to
agree on what work can be done independently and
what work must be done collaboratively. Research
has shown that building such a shared mental
model at the outset of collaborative work
improves efficiency and reduces errors
(Fiore & Schooler, 2004, pp. 140–141).

Too much time gets
spent on issues that
aren't pertinent to you
or your profession.

    What happens when group mem-
bers have different goals? This is not
necessarily a problem if their short-term
goals are compatible and are consistent with
a larger common purpose. Seaburn et al. (1996)
state the following:

> Making the general purpose of any collaboration
> clear often dramatically facilitates the process of weaving short-
> term goals together. Also, making explicit the specific short-term
> goals of each party augers effective progress for those goals. This
> strategy can be very helpful when conflict arises. (p. 52)

When group members have a well-developed understanding of their common purpose, they can maintain the principles of participatory decision making. It is easier to share the reins of leadership when others can be trusted to
do their part toward a common goal.

    Agreeing on group process — how the group works together — is also impor-
tant to building a shared mental model. Being explicit about the group's structure
(e.g., multidisciplinary, interdisciplinary, or transdisciplinary) clarifies expectations for leadership and communication. Agreeing on decision rules increases
engagement, reduces confusion, and helps to prevent needless conflict. Setting

ground rules for communication helps group members meet expectations and maintain the discipline needed for optimal performance. While these agreements may be arrived at informally, documenting them allows new members of a group to grasp the group's shared mental model more quickly and easily.

Healthcare professionals have learned from the experience of other safety-conscious fields such as aviation to reduce the incidence of adverse events by implementing systems for building shared mental models (Burke et al., 2004; Helmreich, 2000). One practical system in template teams is a communication checklist: an instrument designed to prompt discussion among group members about the group's goals and information related to those goals. Lingard et al. (2005) described a research program in which surgical teams designed a pre-operative communication checklist. The purpose of the checklist was to mitigate factors of normal human cognition that contribute to errors by standardizing processes, improving information access, giving feedback, and reducing reliance on memory. Implementation of this checklist significantly reduced communication failures and their consequences (Lingard et al., 2008). As well, members of these surgical teams overwhelmingly agreed that the checklist provided opportunities for team members to "identify and resolve problems and ambiguities" (Lingard et al., 2008, p. 16). The World Health Organization advocates a 19-item surgical safety checklist that has significantly reduced mortality and morbidity around the world (World Health Organization, 2009). These systems approaches to improving patient safety increase the engagement of all group participants and utilize the collective intelligence of the group.

Roles and Boundaries

Open and frank discussion of who does what in the group contributes important detail to its shared mental model. Especially for direct clinical work, group members need clarity about each other's expectations for the following:

- Scope of practice
- Roles: customary functions, including rights, obligations, and expected behavior patterns
- Boundaries: professional or organizational limits to specific actions or functions, as well as limits or bounds to interpersonal relationships

As well, group members need to agree on which duties, functions, and actions are shared among group members and which are unique to certain members of the group. Such agreements prevent wasteful duplication of effort and ensure that all tasks are done by those capable of doing them. This approach minimizes turf wars,

Overlapping roles is hard. It narrows what skills I can practice.

clarifies accountability, and supports ethical behavior. This kind of discussion also ensures that the group has enough people, and the right people, for the job.

As group members negotiate their roles, they need to appreciate each other's training and skill sets and how these distinct backgrounds can lead to conflicting worldviews (Barrow, McKimm, & Gasquoine, 2011; Garman, Leach, & Spector, 2006). As we have seen, self-awareness and good communication are fundamental to making sure that stereotypes or mistaken assumptions do not prevail. Some group members may have to assert themselves, especially those new to the group, those with a new role, or those with capabilities unknown to other group members. It is instructive to consider how one community worked to incorporate a new role into their primary healthcare system:

> ... when the nurse practitioners (NPs) first arrived, they were welcomed by other disciplines and the community, but their role was undefined, and this created some confusion among the physicians, nurse practitioners and public health nurses as to who would be responsible for delivering which services, especially when there was overlap in scopes of practice. A weekend retreat, in which everyone agreed they had a problem and worked together openly and honestly, brought a resolution. As a result of that retreat, guidelines were developed for roles and responsibilities (i.e., who would do what). (Enhancing Interdisciplinary Collaboration in Primary Health Care, n.d., p. 6)

Two factors make it easier for newcomers or those with new roles to step forward: being part of a group that has established a climate of trust and encouragement, and being confident and clear about one's own training and skill set.

Another boundary that needs clarification is that of privacy and confidentiality, especially for patients. On the one hand, patients expect privacy and confidentiality; on the other, they dislike repeating their story unnecessarily and appreciate it when service providers communicate with one another. Most jurisdictions have legal requirements and standards for privacy and confidentiality of health information. Standards and guidelines for confidentiality in clinical work are similar across professions, but some professionals (e.g., social workers, teachers, and psychologists) may regard confidentiality as limiting collaboration more than others (e.g., dietitians, physicians, and physical therapists) (Baerg et al., 2012). In general, patient information is shared on a need-to-know basis between authorized members of the circle of care. Usually, patients are fully informed of how and when information will be shared with other health professionals. Most clinicians find that establishing informed consent for sharing information is an ongoing process. Lynch (2006) advocated developing a sharing information toolkit (e.g., brochures, consent forms, and policy statements) that outlines the roles and responsibilities of each participant in the group. Establishing the limits of confidentiality and information sharing is a good example of how systemic and organizational factors affect interpersonal relationships (Institute for Patient- and Family-Centered Care, 2010b).

EXERCISE 5.1

Consider a patient and a situation familiar for you to answer the following questions:

Who might the patient identify as members of his or her circle of care, people with whom the patient would want to exchange information relevant to the issue at hand?

_____

_____

_____

Which organizations or structures are involved in the care of the patient? Do some have a common chart or automatic access to each other's records?

_____

_____

_____

Are there members within this circle of care who are restricted in their communication; for example, who can receive more information than they can share?

_____

_____

_____

How does current privacy legislation for your jurisdiction affect interprofessional communication?

_____

_____

_____

Principles of privacy and confidentiality also apply to information about colleagues, groups, and organizations. At the interpersonal level, common sense prevails: sensitive personal information about colleagues is disclosed only with their permission. The extent to which information about a group may be shared depends on the nature of the group and may change from time to time. In any case, group members need to be mindful of the consequences of sharing information outside the group. Within larger organizations, there may be restrictions on who can share information outside the organization or across different divisions or levels within the organization. Organizational policies and procedures for sharing information should be readily accessible to all employees.

Resources

One of the most important assets members bring to a group is their knowledge about resources. Resources may range from the local and practical to the systemic and general. Examples of practical local resources include opportunities to interact, time to meet, suitable meeting facilities, synchronized schedules, efficient communication systems, in-house training, local experts, financial backing, and support staff. Examples of general systemic resources include community agencies, funding sources, research reports, online education, and professional initiatives. Timely sharing of knowledge about resources is fundamental to building a shared mental model.

Large organizations often have well-staffed human resources departments that can provide support to working groups. Such support can include help with creating a common vision, team building, communication training, evaluation, quality improvement, and conflict resolution. Such services may also be available through contracts with private sector companies. Third-party support of this type is especially valuable because it allows all group members to participate fully.

Disorganization in the workplace from management or administration makes IPC difficult.

Resources provided by the larger organization can make or break a working group. When organizations provide appropriate resources, working groups can flourish. Insufficient resources can result in dysfunctional groups, where group members may even blame each other for problems that actually arise from organizational or systemic barriers. When groups are struggling, wise leaders consider what resources the group needs, either by reflection, using a self-assessment tool, or engaging an outside

consultant. If the culture of the larger organization or system is not supportive of collaborative work, group members may need to advocate for sufficient
resources. Managers may need to be educated about the value of collaboration and how it can solve problems and provide efficiencies within the larger
organization.

In summary, collaborative work succeeds when competent group members have in common a well-developed mental model of the goals, process,
roles, boundaries, and resources for their work together. The time required
for establishing this shared mental model varies with the purpose, size, and
longevity of the group. A knotwork of clinicians working with an individual
patient and family may require only a few minutes to establish a shared mental model at a meeting or by correspondence. A new clinical or management
team may require dedicated time in meetings or retreats to establish a shared
mental model, which may proceed through several iterations, and may be
reviewed and revised at planned time intervals.

Engagement and Integrity

In his groundbreaking research program where big data meets the social
sciences, Pentland found evidence that "engagement — direct, strong, positive interactions between people — is vital to promoting trustworthy, cooperative behavior" (2014, p. 65). In one study, people in a large community
sample were assigned buddies to encourage them to increase their physical
activity. After analyzing gigabytes of contextual data, the researchers found
that the number of positive interactions people had with their buddies pre-
dicted not only their expressions of trust in each other, but also increased
physical activity, even after the experiment ended (pp. 66–69). In other
words, engagement was related to the quality of relationships and to sustained behavior change.

In another study, Pentland (2014, pp. 87–89) reported that performance
on a group IQ test was not related to measures of cohesion, motivation, or
satisfaction, but rather to group process. Groups with a few people who
dominated the conversation were collectively less intelligent than were those
groups with an equal distribution of conversation. More specifically, the most
successful groups had a large number of diverse ideas, with dense interactions characterized by short contributions and briefer responses that served
to validate or invalidate ideas and build consensus. In other words, Pentland's
research indicated that the intelligence, personality, and skill of individual
group members mattered less to the success of their group than the pattern of
the flow of ideas.

Taking the results of these and other studies together, Pentland (2014)
concluded that engagement builds a culture of cooperation and improves

the collective intelligence of the group. Applying these research results to collaborative patient- and family-centered healthcare, we can see how the collective intelligence of the group depends on the principles of participatory decision making: full participation, mutual understanding, inclusive solutions, and shared responsibility. Pentland noted that engagement must be between all the members of a group, not just between the individual and the group (as in a group meeting) or between the individual and the leader of the group. Repeated positive interactions form the foundation for trust, which is essentially an expectation of future cooperative behavior (2014, pp. 76–78).

EXERCISE 5.2

Reflect on the engagement and pattern of flow of ideas in a group in which you have participated and answer the following questions:

Were there group members who did not seem engaged?

_____

_____

_____

How did this affect the performance of the group?

_____

_____

_____

What factors might have contributed to the apparent lack of engagement of those group members?

_____

_____

_____

Individual integrity also contributes to trust and cooperative behavior among group members. Burbules (1993) identified a set of virtues that contribute to integrity in leadership. We have taken this list and arranged them to form the mnemonic *crash a lot*. We suggest that developing expertise in interprofessional collaboration is like mastering snowboarding or cycling: crashing from time to time is to be expected.

- Concern for others and the problem
- Respect for differences
- Appreciating others' contributions and skills
- Sharing openly with all
- Hoping for outcomes not achievable alone
- Affection and caring for group members
- Learning from each other
- Owning your responsibilities
- Trusting others and the process

This list of virtues should be familiar to you by now, but the term *affection* merits some additional discussion. While affection for other group members is not required, it frequently takes root when group members interact frequently, cooperatively, and with integrity and respect. The word *respect* derives from Latin, meaning to "see again." When group members interact enough to see each other in a new light, they reduce stereotypes and prevent mistaken assumptions that can inhibit or derail group process.

Assessment and Evaluation

Assessment and evaluation are important to any professional endeavor, whether through informal processes such as individual self-reflection or through formal processes such as quality-improvement cycles, performance reviews, and accreditation. Evaluation can serve one or more functions:

- Measuring effectiveness
- Identifying strengths and successes
- Identifying areas for improvement
- Strengthening relationships through the very process of evaluation

The focus of evaluation of collaborative work may center on outcomes, process, or both. For example, group members may choose to measure desired outcomes (e.g., increased accessibility to services) or an aspect of group functioning (e.g., giving feedback). Assessment methods may range from audits of existing data (e.g., patient records) to comprehensive systematic reviews using observation, questionnaires, self-study, and/or interviews. The extent to which clinical healthcare teams are patient and family centered can be measured by their decisions and outcomes (e.g., treatment plans). In this section, we present a brief guide to evaluation of collaborative work at individual and organizational levels, with an emphasis on self-study and reflection.

Individuals

At an individual level, performance reviews and trainee evaluation systems may or may not include items or sections that assess interprofessional collaboration skills and competencies. Those who wish to update their local assessment measures will find it helpful to review one or more of the following competency frameworks. In the United States, the document "Core Competencies for Interprofessional Collaborative Practice" (Interprofessional Education Collaborative Expert Panel, 2011) identifies competencies in four domains: values/ethics for interprofessional practice, roles/responsibilities, interprofessional communication, and teams and teamwork. In Canada, the "National Interprofessional Competency Framework" (Canadian Interprofessional Health Collaborative, 2010) has four slightly different domains: role clarification, team functioning, interprofessional conflict resolution, and collaborative leadership. In the United Kingdom, the four domains identified by the Interprofessional Education Team at Sheffield Hallam University (2010) are collaborative working, reflection, cultural awareness and ethical practice, and organizational competence. While these three frameworks differ somewhat in the competencies included and how they are defined and organized, they are useful resources for descriptions of individual competencies for interprofessional collaboration.

For individuals with high levels of self-awareness and deep appreciation of the competencies required for successful collaboration, self-reflection can be useful. Unfortunately, many individuals overestimate their performance on social or intellectual tasks, especially poorer performers who lack insight into their shortcomings because they are not aware of the competencies needed for skilled performance (Ehrlinger, Johnson, Banner, Dunning, & Kruger, 2008; Kruger & Dunning, 1999). As Dave Barry noted, we all think we are above average drivers (1998, p. 182). Fortunately, research indicates that individuals can achieve more realistic self-appraisals after receiving training on the skills needed for a task (Kruger & Dunning, 1999). For this reason, practicing professionals, especially those not subject to peer review,

EXERCISE 5.3

The following competency frameworks are available online. Compare them with the principles, standards, or competencies for interprofessional collaboration for your own profession, institution, or organization:

Core Competencies for Interprofessional Collaborative Practice, Report of an Expert Panel, 2011: www.aacn.nche.edu/education-resources/ipecreport.pdf

A National Interprofessional Competency Framework, Canadian Interprofessional Health Collaborative, 2010: www.cihc.ca/files /CIHC_IPCompetencies_Feb1210.pdf

Interprofessional Capability Framework 2010, Mini-Guide, Sheffield Hallam University: www.health.heacademy.ac.uk/doc/resources/icf2010 .pdf/view.html

How do the competencies in these frameworks compare with those of your own profession, institution, or organization? What do they have in common? What is missing?

_____

_____

_____

_____

_____

_____

_____

_____

_____

_____

_____

should take advantage of opportunities to update their knowledge and skills for interprofessional collaboration in order to monitor their competencies in this area more accurately.

Groups, Teams, and Systems

Evaluating collaborative practice in healthcare at the organizational level can be a daunting task; fortunately, some excellent guides and resources are available. Heinemann and Zeiss (2002) used a conceptual model of team performance in healthcare to organize a comprehensive review of assessment instruments ranging from focused to broad spectrum. Rosen et al. presented a "practical guide to navigating the complexities of designing and implementing a team performance measurement system within the context of a healthcare safety and quality improvement initiative" (2013, p. 59). Some recently published research tools include the Assessment of Interprofessional Team Collaboration Scale (Orchard, King, Khalili, & Bezzina, 2012) and the Interprofessional Socialization and Valuing Scale (King, Shaw, Orchard, & Miller, 2010).

When it works well, it's a beautiful thing. When it doesn't work well, things can get really ugly.

While some groups may undergo externally initiated evaluation (e.g., initiated by management), other groups may choose to evaluate themselves. The process of reflection can offer valuable insights (Margalef García & Pareja Roblin, 2008; Reeves & Freeth, 2006). Rodgers (2002) stated that effective reflection is rooted in the tradition of scientific inquiry and, therefore, should be conducted in a spirit of openness to ensure intellectual growth and development. Rodgers also noted that when members of a community engage in reflection interactively, they move from one experience to the next with a deeper understanding of the interconnections of their experiences and ideas.

Self-study, a form of structured reflection, has been used extensively in the field of education for pedagogical and practice-related purposes (Louie, Drevdahl, Purdy, & Stackman, 2003). The following steps are typical for this kind of self-study:

- Identify the group's goals for the exercise.
- Employ an experienced external facilitator.
- Together with the facilitator, develop a series of questions for the self-study exercise.
- Under the guidance of the facilitator, discuss the questions as a group.

- Document group members' responses to the questions, either during the discussion or by transcribing an audio/video recording of the discussion.
- Extract key themes from the documentation. Provide a written account of these themes to group members.

This qualitative approach to self-study can help a group decide how to proceed, for example, by pinpointing areas for education or professional development. By identifying the challenges that have been overcome, groups can celebrate their successes.

With the help of an external facilitator, the authors participated in a self-study early in their partnership. The facilitator generated a list of evaluation questions, some of which were adapted from the Wilder Collaboration Factors Inventory (Mattessich, Murray-Close, & Monsey, 2001). We offer these questions in Appendix D for those who may find them useful in generating their own questions for self-study.

Some groups may find it workable to have one of their own members act as a facilitator for a straightforward self-study experience, such as reflecting on specific questions provided by an accrediting body to meet accreditation requirements. Experienced external facilitators are especially valuable when there are complex questions, unclear goals, or internal unresolved conflict. Facilitators experienced with leading appreciative inquiry — asking individuals to describe their best experience with collaboration — can help new working groups build a shared mental model, or help established groups stuck in paradoxical dilemmas (Bushe, 1998).

For a quantitative approach to self-study, we offer a 20-item survey called the Collaboration Self-Assessment Tool (CSAT) that can be used to check on the vital signs of a working group (see Appendix E). This survey loosely follows the framework presented in this book. The first six items of the CSAT ask raters to consider the shared mental model of the group as well as organizational and systemic factors that affect group functioning. Items 7 through 11 deal with communication and engagement. Items 12 through 15 address decision making, leadership, and mutual understanding of roles and responsibilities. The last five items ask for ratings of the group's efficacy and personal feelings about participating in the group.

To analyze the results of the CSAT, look for patterns. For some items, there may be a high level of agreement among group members, in a positive or negative direction. For other items, there may be a high degree of variance among group members' responses, with some members responding differently from the majority of the group. Group members benefit from seeing both the aggregated results as well as the variation, especially when there are outliers. Presenting the pattern of results both ways allows groups to decide on their priorities for focused discussion, intervention, or additional training.

WEAVING THE FABRIC OF COLLABORATION

When the CSAT is used to track changes in a group's vital signs over time, it is important to celebrate the group's successes in addition to focusing on areas for improvement.

Applying the Framework

The framework presented in this book can also be a useful tool for reflection and problem solving (see Table 5.1). The themes shown in Table 5.1 represent the core issues of the vignettes described throughout this book, but there are many potential themes for each of the cells of this framework — you have been invited to add more themes at the end of chapters 2, 3, and 4. To apply this framework in real-world situations, individuals or groups may choose to focus on a cell, row, or column of this framework to identify areas for ongoing development. Problem solving may be aided by using the framework to identify where the weakness or breakdown is occurring: in which competency domain or domains, at what level or levels of interaction. The framework provides a reminder that it is important to be cognizant of the organizational and systemic context of your working group, even when focusing primarily on interpersonal processes.

TABLE 5.1 FRAMEWORK

	INTERPERSONAL	ORGANIZATIONAL	SYSTEMIC
Teamwork	Respect Your examples:	Group structure Your examples:	Population changes Your examples:

Leadership	Participatory decision
	  making
	Your examples:
		Conflict about
		  resources
		  and procedures
		Your examples:
			Conflict about
			  scope of
			  practice
			Your examples:

Communication	Mutual understanding Your examples:	Timeliness Your examples:	Stereotypes Your examples:

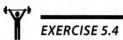

EXERCISE 5.4

Consider the following brief descriptions of situations in healthcare and identify where they best fit in the framework, keeping in mind that they might exemplify more than one cell. Think of some other examples of situations to map into this framework.

Public health services struggle to provide culturally appropriate services to an expanding immigrant community.

_____

_____

A new member of a long-standing and tightly knit team questions the existing structure of the team.

_____

_____

Mental health practitioners adapt to an amalgamation of two agencies into one.

_____

_____

Frontline service providers learn to use a new electronic charting system.

_____

_____

A surgical unit trains and requires members of its teams to use a communication checklist before each operation.

_____

_____

Add your own examples:

_____

_____

In this final chapter, we have outlined important components of collaboration in healthcare. For collaboration to work, participants need a shared mental model of their goals, processes, roles, boundaries, and resources. Participants need to engage in collaboration with optimism and integrity. A variety of methods and tools can be used to evaluate interprofessional collaboration so that individuals and groups are accountable for their actions. Applying the competencies of teamwork, leadership, and communication at all levels of engagement allows members of a collaborative working group to lead each other to successful achievement of their goals, following a mutually agreed upon process, resolving differences, evaluating outcomes, and celebrating successes.

Closing Words

> It is hardly possible to overrate the value . . . of placing human beings in contact with persons dissimilar to themselves, and with modes of thought and action unlike those with which they are familiar. . . . Such communication has always been, and is peculiarly in the present age, one of the primary sources of progress.
>
> —John Stuart Mill, 1848

Mill's words about the value of diversity to progress in human endeavors seem as relevant today as they were more than 160 years ago. We enlarge our vision and expand our capacity by connecting with others who think and behave differently. When we capitalize on the synergy of interprofessional collaboration in healthcare, we generate better outcomes and feel more satisfied with our work at the same time.

Collaborating is like weaving. Weavers place guiding threads (the warp) on a frame or loom and then weave visible threads (the weft) over and under the warp. The daily actions and outcomes of interprofessional collaboration are the visible threads, while competencies of the participants — their attitudes, beliefs, values, knowledge, and skills — are the hidden guiding threads on which the fabric of collaboration is woven. We hope that this book provides you with a framework, or loom, for weaving. The texture and design of your collaboration will be infinitely variable depending on the setting, participants, and goals. In each case, you strengthen the fabric by constructing a shared mental model, engaging with others, behaving with integrity, and applying your competencies for teamwork, leadership, and communication.

Appendix A
Attitudes toward Health Care Teams Scale[1]

Circle one number for each statement.

	STRONGLY DISAGREE	MODERATELY DISAGREE	SOMEWHAT DISAGREE	SOMEWHAT AGREE	MODERATELY AGREE	STRONGLY AGREE
1	Working on teams unnecessarily complicates things most of the time.	1	2	3	4	5	6
2	The team approach improves the quality of care to patients.	1	2	3	4	5	6
3	Team meetings foster communication among team members from different disciplines.	1	2	3	4	5	6
4	Physicians have the right to alter patient care plans developed by the team.	1	2	3	4	5	6
5	Patients receiving team care are more likely than other patients to be treated as whole persons.	1	2	3	4	5	6
6	A team's primary purpose is to assist physicians in achieving treatment goals for patients.	1	2	3	4	5	6
7	Working on a team keeps most health professionals enthusiastic and interested in their jobs.	1	2	3	4	5	6
8	Patients are less satisfied with their care when it is provided by a team.	1	2	3	4	5	6
9	Developing a patient care plan with other team members avoids errors in delivering care.	1	2	3	4	5	6
10	When developing interdisciplinary patient care plans, much time is wasted translating jargon from other disciplines.	1	2	3	4	5	6

(Continued)

		STRONGLY DISAGREE	MODERATELY DISAGREE	SOMEWHAT DISAGREE	SOMEWHAT AGREE	MODERATELY AGREE	STRONGLY AGREE
11.	Health professionals working on teams are more responsive than others to the emotional and financial needs of patients.	1	2	3	4	5	6
12.	Developing an interdisciplinary patient care plan is excessively time consuming.	1	2	3	4	5	6
13.	The physician should not always have the final word in decisions made by health care teams.	1	2	3	4	5	6
14.	The give and take among team members helps them to make better patient care decisions.	1	2	3	4	5	6
15.	In most instances, the time required for team meetings could be better spent in other ways.	1	2	3	4	5	6
16.	The physician has the ultimate legal responsibility for decisions made by the team.	1	2	3	4	5	6
17.	Hospital patients who receive team care are better prepared for discharge than other patients.	1	2	3	4	5	6
18.	Physicians are natural team leaders.	1	2	3	4	5	6
19.	The team approach makes the delivery of care more efficient.	1	2	3	4	5	6
20.	The team approach permits health professionals to meet the needs of family caregivers as well as patients.	1	2	3	4	5	6
21.	Having to report observations to the team helps team members better understand the work of other health professionals.	1	2	3	4	5	6

NOTE

1 Hyer, K., Fairchild, S., Abraham, I., Mezey, M., & Fulmer, T. (2000). Measuring attitudes related to interdisciplinary training: Revisiting the Heinemann, Schmitt and Farrell "Attitudes toward health care teams" scale. *Journal of Interprofessional Care, 14*, 249–258.

Appendix B
Shared Leadership Behavior Checklist

CATEGORY	TYPE OF BEHAVIOR	✔ EACH TIME THIS BEHAVIOR OCCURS	NOTES
Group task	**Initiating:** proposing goals, setting agendas, defining problems, suggesting solutions, developing plans		
	Seeking information: asking for facts, information, opinions, ideas and feelings		
	Giving information: offering facts, information, opinions, ideas and feelings		
	Clarifying/Elaborating: interpreting ideas, clearing up confusions, defining terms, indicating alternatives, giving examples		
	Summarizing: restating or pulling together related ideas		
	Consensus testing: offering a conclusion to see if the group agrees		
	Evaluating: examining the feasibility/rightness of ideas, evaluating alternatives, comparing group decisions with group standards and goals		
	Recording: ensuring that a written record is made of group ideas, decisions, and plans		
Group building and maintenance	**Harmonizing:** reconcilling disagreements, reducing tension (by using humor, suggesting breaks, offering fun approaches to work)		
	Gatekeeping and trust building: encouraging everyone to participate, demonstrating acceptance and openness to the ideas of others, encouraging individuality, promoting open discussion of conflicts		
	Supporting and encouraging: being friendly, warm, and responsive (in speech, gesture, facial expression), giving recognition for contributions		
	Compromising: admitting error, shifting position in response to new insights		
	Coordinating and regulating: drawing together activities of members or subgroups, influencing the direction and tempo of the group's work		

Appendix C
Active Listening Checklist

Do you think the people not talking (the listeners) are actually listening? What are the signs that make you think that? Consider, do they...

CATEGORY	TYPE OF BEHAVIOR	✔ IF YOU OBSERVE THIS BEHAVIOR	NOTES
Nonverbal behavior	Mirror the speaker's posture (e.g., sit down if speaker is sitting)		
	Lean forward		
	Face the speaker (e.g., have their feet pointing toward the speaker)		
	Make consistent eye contact		
	Change facial expressions (i.e., face not frozen)		
	Have arms uncrossed		
	Keep a reasonable distance from the person, to allow for ease of conversation		
	Make efforts to limit distractions (e.g., close door, ignore phone, turn away from window)		
	Convey nonverbal signals that are consistent with verbal messages		
Verbal behavior	Avoid interrupting to take over the speaker role		
	Use interjections (e.g., "oh," "right")		
	Ask questions to clarify		
	Paraphrase or summarize the speaker's message		
	Reflect the speaker's feelings, where appropriate		

Appendix D
Structured Group Reflection Questions[1]

1. Please summarize the work you have done and what you feel your group has accomplished.
2. Please share a time when you were part of another collaborative experience. Looking back at that experience:
   - What made the team functional?
   - What was your contribution?
   - What did you learn about teams from that experience?
   - What did you learn about yourself?
   - What did you value about others?
3. What has worked well in this collaboration? What were the positives?
4. What incentives were present for you during the project?
5. What challenges did you encounter?
6. What did you learn from this group experience?
7. Consider the value of this experience and the contributions of each group member.
   - What unique skills, strengths, or assets did you bring to the group?
   - What assets do you value in the other members of your group?
8. What organizations supported your efforts and how?
9. What does collaboration mean to you?
10. What logistics were in place in order for you to accomplish your goals?
11. What was your least favorite experience during this project?
12. What barriers did you experience?
13. What were your strategies for addressing the barriers? Did they work? Why or why not?
14. Was conflict acknowledged and processed?

15. If you could wave a magic wand and conjure three gifts that would help this team be its very best, what gifts would you wish for?

16. Any closing comments? Anything else you would like to share about your experience?

NOTE
1 C. Zukewich, personal communication, 2007.

Appendix E
Collaboration Self-Assessment Tool (CSAT)

	COLLABORATION SELF-ASSESSMENT TOOL (CSAT)	STRONGLY DISAGREE	MODERATELY DISAGREE	SOMEWHAT DISAGREE	SOMEWHAT AGREE	MODERATELY AGREE	STRONGLY AGREE
1	We have a clear understanding of our goals.	1	2	3	4	5	6
2	We have shared values.	1	2	3	4	5	6
3	We have the right organizational structure to meet our goals.	1	2	3	4	5	6
4	We have sufficient resources to meet our goals.	1	2	3	4	5	6
5	We provide patient- and family-centered care.	1	2	3	4	5	6
6	Patients/Families/Clients know what to expect from us.	1	2	3	4	5	6
7	We all express ourselves openly, honestly, and directly.	1	2	3	4	5	6
8	We all listen carefully to each other.	1	2	3	4	5	6
9	We all are sensitive to the needs of our group.	1	2	3	4	5	6
10	We all participate actively in our group.	1	2	3	4	5	6
11	We have a climate of mutual trust where the atmosphere is friendly and relaxed.	1	2	3	4	5	6
12	Leadership is shared among us according to our abilities and insights.	1	2	3	4	5	6

COLLABORATION SELF-ASSESSMENT TOOL (CSAT)	STRONGLY DISAGREE	MODERATELY DISAGREE	SOMEWHAT DISAGREE	SOMEWHAT AGREE	MODERATELY AGREE	STRONGLY AGREE
13 We each support the final decision, even when it was not our idea.	1	2	3	4	5	6
14 Everyone else understands my role and responsibilities.	1	2	3	4	5	6
15 I understand everyone else's role and responsibilities.	1	2	3	4	5	6
16 Our productivity is high.	1	2	3	4	5	6
17 Our meetings follow the agenda and start and end on time.	1	2	3	4	5	6
18 We make decisions in a timely manner.	1	2	3	4	5	6
19 I feel like a valued member of our group.	1	2	3	4	5	6
20 Overall, I am satisfied with my participation in our group.	1	2	3	4	5	6

References

Accreditation Canada. (2014). *Required organizational practices handbook 2014.* Retrieved from www.accreditation.ca/sites/default/files/rop-handbook-2014-en.pdf

Agency for Healthcare Research and Quality. (2014). *Patient safety primers: Teamwork training.* Retrieved from psnet.ahrq.gov/primer.aspx?primerID=5

AIPHE (Accreditation of Interprofessional Health Education). (2011). *Interprofessional health education accreditation standards guide.* Retrieved from www.cihc.ca/files/resources/public/English/AIPHE%20Interprofessional%20Health%20Education%20Accreditation%20Standards%20Guide_EN.pdf

Alonso, A., & Dunleavy, D. M. (2013). Building teamwork skills in healthcare: The case for communication and coordination competencies. In E. Salas & K. Frush (with D. P. Baker, J. B. Battles, H. B. King, & R. L. Wears) (Eds.), Improving patient safety through teamwork and team training (pp. 41–58). New York, NY: Oxford University Press.

American Nurses Association/American Organization of Nurse Executives (n.d.). *Principles for collaborative relationships between clinical nurses and nurse managers.* Retrieved from www.nursingworld.org/MainMenuCategories/ThePracticeofProfessionalNursing/NursingStandards/ANAPrinciples/Principles-of-Collaborative-Relationships.pdf

Artis, A. B. (2008). Improving marketing students' reading comprehension with the SQ3R method. *Journal of Marketing Education, 30*(2), 130–137. http://dx.doi.org/10.1177/0273475308318070

Avery, C. (2001). *Teamwork is an individual skill.* San Francisco, CA: Berrett-Koehler.

Baerg, K., Lake, D., & Paslawski, T. (2012). Survey of interprofessional collaboration learning needs and training interest in health professionals, teachers, and students: An exploratory study. *Journal of Research in Interprofessional Practice and Education, 2,* 187–204. Retrieved from www.jripe.org/jripe/index.php/journal/article/viewArticle/47

Barrow, M., McKimm, J., & Gasquoine, S. (2011). The policy and the practice: Early-career doctors and nurses as leaders and followers in the delivery of health care. *Advances in Health Sciences Education : Theory and Practice, 16*(1), 17–29. http://dx.doi.org/10.1007/s10459-010-9239-2

Barry, D. (1998). *Dave Barry turns 50.* New York, NY: Ballantine.

Barry, M. J., & Edgman-Levitan, S. (2012). Shared decision making: The pinnacle of patient-centered care. *New England Journal of Medicine, 366*(9), 780–781. http://dx.doi.org/10.1056/NEJMp1109283

Bass, B. M. (1990). *Bass & Stogdill's handbook of leadership: Theory, research, and management applications* (3rd ed.). New York, NY: The Free Press.

Beebe, S. A., Beebe, S. J., Redmond, M. V., & Geerinck, T. M. (2004). *Interpersonal communication: Relating to others.* Toronto, ON: Pearson Education Canada.

Benne, K. D., & Sheats, P. (1948). Functional roles of group members. *Journal of Social Issues, 4,* 41–49. Republished in 2007 in *Group Facilitation: A Research & Applications Journal, 8,* 30–35. Retrieved from www.iaf-world.org/Libraries/IAF_Journals/Functional_Roles_of_Group_Members.sflb.ashx

Bennis, W. G., & Nanus, B. (1997). *Leaders: Strategies for taking charge* (2nd ed.). New York, NY: HarperBusiness.

Boone, K. W. (2011). *The CDA™ Book*. New York, NY: Springer.

Borrell-Carrio, F., Suchman, A. L., & Epstein, R. M. (2004). The biopsychosocial model 25 years later: Principles, practice, and scientific inquiry. *Annals of Family Medicine, 2*(6), 576–582. http://dx.doi.org/10.1370/afm.245

Burbules, N. C. (1993). *Dialogue in teaching: Theory and practice*. New York, NY: Teachers College.

Burke, C. S., Salas, E., Wilson-Donnelly, K., & Priest, H. (2004). How to turn a team of experts into an expert medical team: Guidance from the aviation and military communities. *Quality & Safety in Health Care, 13*(suppl_1), i96–i104. Retrieved from qualitysafety.bmj.com/. http://dx.doi.org/10.1136/qshc.2004.009829

Bushe, G. R. (1998). Appreciative inquiry with teams. *Organization Development Journal, 16*(3), 41–50.

Canadian Interprofessional Health Collaborative. (2009). *What is collaborative practice?* Retrieved from www.cihc.ca/files/CIHC_Factsheets_CP_Feb09.pdf

Canadian Interprofessional Health Collaborative. (2010). *A national interprofessional health competency framework*. Retrieved from www.cihc.ca/files/CIHC_IPCompetencies_Feb1210.pdf

Canadian Medical Protective Association. (February 2008). *Collaborative care: A medical liability perspective*. Retrieved from https://oplfrpd5.cmpa-acpm.ca/safety/-/asset_publisher/N6oEDMrzRbCC/content/collaborative-ca-1

Carpenter, J. (1995). Doctors and nurses: Stereotypes and stereotype change in interprofessional education. *Journal of Interprofessional Care, 9*(2), 151–161. http://dx.doi.org/10.3109/13561829509047849

Cegala, D. J., & Lenzmeier Broz, S. (2002). Physician communication skills training: A review of theoretical backgrounds, objectives and skills. *Medical Education, 36*(11), 1004–1016. http://dx.doi.org/10.1046/j.1365-2923.2002.01331.x

Chandler, D. (2007). *Semiotics: The basics* (2nd ed.). New York, NY: Routledge.

Chant, S., Jenkinson, T., Randle, J., Russell, G., & Webb, C. (2002). Communication skills training in healthcare: A review of the literature. *Nurse Education Today, 22*(3), 189–202. http://dx.doi.org/10.1054/nedt.2001.0690

Chidambaram, L., & Bostrom, R. (1997). Group development: A review and synthesis of developmental models. *Group Decision and Negotiation, 6*(2), 159–187. http://dx.doi.org/10.1023/A:1008603328241

Clark, P. (1997). Values in health care professional socialization: Implications for geriatric education in interdisciplinary teamwork. *Gerontologist, 37*(4), 441–451. http://dx.doi.org/10.1093/geront/37.4.441

Conference Board of Canada. (April 2007). *Liability risks in interdisciplinary care: Thinking outside the box*. Retrieved from www.caot.ca/pdfs/Liability%20Risks%20report.pdf

Cragan, J. F., & Wright, D. W. (1999). *Communication in small groups: Theory, process and skills*. Belmont, CA: Wadsworth.

Curley, C., McEachern, J. E., & Speroff, T. (1998). A firm trial of interdisciplinary rounds on the inpatient medical wards: An intervention designed using continuous quality improvement. *Medical Care, 36*(8), AS4–AS12. Retrieved from www.jstor.org/stable/3767037

D'Amour, D., & Oandasan, I. (2005). Interprofessionality as the field of interprofessional practice and interprofessional education: An emerging concept. *Journal of Interprofessional Care, 19*(s1 Suppl. 1), 8–20. http://dx.doi.org/10.1080/13561820500081604

De Meester, K., Verspuy, M., Monsieurs, K. G., & Van Bogaert, P. (2013). SBAR improves nurse–physician communication and reduces unexpected death: A pre and post intervention study. *Resuscitation, 84*(9), 1192–1196. http://dx.doi.org/10.1016/j.resuscitation.2013.03.016

Dobie, S. (2007). Reflections on a well-traveled path: Self-awareness, mindful practice, and relationship-centered care as foundations for medical education. *Academic Medicine, 82*(4), 422–427. http://dx.doi.org/10.1097/01.ACM.0000259374.52323.62

Doyle, M. E., & Smith, M. K. (2001a). Classical leadership. *The encyclopedia of informal education.* Retrieved from www.infed.org/leadership/traditional_leadership.htm

Doyle, M. E., & Smith, M. K. (2001b). Shared leadership. *The encyclopedia of informal education.* Retrieved from www.infed.org/leadership/shared_leadership.htm

Duffy, F. D., Gordon, G. H., Whelan, G., Cole-Kelly, K., & Frankel, R. (2004). Assessing competence in communication and interpersonal skills: The Kalamazoo II report. *Academic Medicine, 79*(6), 495–507. http://dx.doi.org/10.1097/00001888-200406000-00002

Ehrlinger, J., Johnson, K., Banner, M., Dunning, D., & Kruger, J. (2008). Why the unskilled are unaware: Further explorations of (absent) self-insight among the incompetent. *Organizational Behavior and Human Decision Processes, 105*(1), 98–121. http://dx.doi.org/10.1016/j.obhdp.2007.05.002

Enhancing Interdisciplinary Collaboration in Primary Health Care. (n.d.). *Interdisciplinary primary health care: Finding the answers: A case study report.* Retrieved from www.eicp.ca/en/toolkit/EICP-Case-Studies-Report-Final-Aug-14.pdf

Farahani, M. A., Sahragard, R., Caroll, J. K., & Mohammadi, E. (2011). Communication barriers to patient education in cardiac inpatient care: A qualitative study of multiple perspectives. *International Journal of Nursing Practice, 17*(3), 322–328. http://dx.doi.org/10.1111/j.1440-172X.2011.01940.x

Fay, N., Page, A. C., & Serfaty, C. (2010). Listeners influence speakers' perceived communication effectiveness. *Journal of Experimental Social Psychology, 46*(4), 689–692. http://dx.doi.org/10.1016/j.jesp.2010.02.012

Fiore, S. M., & Schooler, J. W. (2004). Process mapping and shared cognition: Teamwork and the development of shared problem models. In E. Salas & S. M. Fiore (Eds.), *Team cognition: Understanding the factors that drive process and performance* (pp. 133–152). Washington, DC: American Psychological Association. http://dx.doi.org/10.1037/10690-007

Fiske, S. T. (1998). Stereotyping, prejudice, and discrimination. In D. T. Gilbert, S. T. Fiske, & G. Lindzey (Eds.), *The handbook of social psychology* (4th ed., Vol. 2, pp. 357–411). New York, NY: McGraw-Hill.

Fletcher, J. K., & Käufer, K. (2003). Shared leadership: Paradox and possibility. In C. L. Pearce & J. A. Conger (Eds.), *Shared leadership: Reframing the hows and whys of leadership* (pp. 21–47). Thousand Oaks, CA: Sage. http://dx.doi.org/10.4135/9781452229539.n2

Foley, G. M. (1990). Portrait of the arena evaluation: Assessment in the transdisciplinary approach. In E. D. Gibbs & D. M. Teti (Eds.), *Interdisciplinary assessment of infants: A guide for early intervention professionals* (pp. 271–286). Baltimore, MD: Paul H. Brookes.

Frenk, J., Chen, L., Bhutta, Z.A., et al. (2010). Health professionals for a new century: Transforming education to strengthen health systems in an interdependent world. *Lancet, 376*(9756), 1923–1958. http://dx.doi.org/10.1016/S0140-6736(10)61854-5

Fuertes, J. N., Potere, J. C., & Ramirez, K. Y. (2002). Effects of speech accents on interpersonal evaluations: Implications for counseling practice and research. *Cultural Diversity & Ethnic Minority Psychology, 8*(4), 346–356. http://dx.doi.org/10.1037/1099-9809.8.4.347

Garman, A. N., Leach, D. C., & Spector, N. (2006). Worldviews in collision: Conflict and collaboration across professional lines. *Journal of Organizational Behavior, 27*(7), 829–849. http://dx.doi.org/10.1002/job.394

General Dental Council. (2011). *Standards for the dental team.* Retrieved from www.gdc-uk.org/Newsandpublications/Publications/Publications/Standards%20for%20the%20Dental%20Team.pdf

Gilbert, E., Ussher, J. M., Perz, J., Hobbs, K., & Kirsten, L. (2010). Positive and negative interactions with health professionals: A qualitative investigation of the experiences of informal cancer carers. *Cancer Nursing, 33*(6), E1–E9. http://dx.doi.org/10.1097/NCC.0b013e3181da365d

Givens, D. B. (2015). *The nonverbal dictionary of gestures, signs and body cues*. Spokane, WA: Center for Nonverbal Studies Press. Retrieved from center-for-nonverbal-studies.org/6101.html

Gottesdiener, E. (2002). *Requirements by collaboration: Workshops for defining needs*. Boston, MA: Pearson Education.

Grice, H. P. (1975). Logic and conversation. In P. Cole & J. L. Morgan (Eds.), Syntax and semantics (Vol. 3). *Speech acts* (pp. 41–58). New York, NY: Seminar.

Hackman, J. R. (1990). *Groups that work (and those that don't): Creating conditions for effective teamwork*. San Francisco, CA: Jossey-Bass.

Haig, K. M., Sutton, S., & Whittington, J. (2006). SBAR: A shared mental model for improving communication between clinicians. *Joint Commission Journal on Quality and Patient Safety, 32,* 167–175.

Harnack, R. V., Fest, T. B., & Jones, B. S. (1977). *Group discussion: Theory and technique*. Englewood Cliffs, NJ: Prentice-Hall.

Hartrick Doane, G., Stajduhar, K., Causton, E., Bidgood, D., & Cox, A. (2012). End-of-life care and interprofessional communication: Not simply a matter of "more." *Health and Interprofessional Practice, 1*(3). http://dx.doi.org/10.7772/2159-1253.1028

Hawkins, P., & Shohet, R. (2006). *Supervision in the helping professions* (3rd ed.). Berkshire, UK: Open University Press.

Heinemann, G. D., Schmitt, M. H., Farrell, M. P., & Brallier, S. A. (1999). Development of an attitudes toward health care teams scale. *Evaluation & the Health Professions, 22*(1), 123–142. http://dx.doi.org/10.1177/01632789922034202

Heinemann, G. D. & Zeiss, A. M. (Eds.). (2002). *Team performance in health care: Assessment and development*. New York, NY: Kluwer Academic. http://dx.doi.org/10.1007/978-1-4615-0581-5

Helmreich, R. L. (2000). On error: Lessons from aviation. *BMJ: British Medical Journal, 320*(7237), 781–785. Retrieved from www.jstor.org/stable/25187424

Ho, K. (2008). The synergy of interprofessional collaboration and social accountability: Their multiplying effects. *Journal of Interprofessional Care, 22*(s1), 1–3. http://dx.doi.org/10.1080/13561820802013370

Hosman, L. (1989). The evaluative consequences of hedges, hesitations, and intensifiers: Powerful and powerless speech styles. *Human Communication Research, 15*(3), 383–406. http://dx.doi.org/10.1111/j.1468-2958.1989.tb00190.x

Hyer, K., Fairchild, S., Abraham, I., Mezey, M., & Fulmer, T. (2000). Measuring attitudes related to interdisciplinary training: Revisiting the Heinemann, Schmitt and Farrell "Attitudes toward health care teams" scale. *Journal of Interprofessional Care, 14*(3), 249–258. http:// doi:10.1080/jic.14.3.249.258

Institute for Healthcare Improvement. (n.d.). *SBAR Toolkit*. Retrieved from www.ihi.org/resources/Pages/Tools/SBARToolkit.aspx

Institute for Patient- and Family-Centered Care. (2010a). *What are the core concepts of patient- and family-centered care?* Retrieved from www.ipfcc.org/faq.html

Institute for Patient- and Family-Centered Care. (2010b). *HIPAA: Providing new opportunities for collaboration*. Retrieved from www.ipfcc.org/advance/hipaa.pdf

Interprofessional Education Collaborative Expert Panel. (2011). *Core competencies for interprofessional collaborative practice: Report of an expert panel*. Washington, DC: Interprofessional Education Collaborative. Retrieved from www.aacn.nche.edu/education-resources/ipecreport.pdf

Interprofessional Education Team. (2010). *Interprofessional capability framework 2010 mini-guide*. Sheffield Hallam University. Retrieved from www.health.heacademy.ac.uk/doc/resources/icf2010.pdf/view.html

Ipe, M. (2003). Knowledge sharing in organizations: A conceptual framework. *Human Resource Development Review, 2*(4), 337–359. http://dx.doi.org/10.1177/1534484303257985

Iyer, P. (2014). *The art of stillness: Adventures in going nowhere*. New York, NY: Simon and Schuster/TED.

Joint Commission. (2013). *Comprehensive accreditation manual for hospitals*. Oakbrook Terrace, IL: The Joint Commission.

Kaner, S. (with Lind, L., Toldi, C., Fisk, S., & Berger, D.). (2007). *Facilitator's guide to participatory decision-making* (2nd ed.). San Francisco, CA: Jossey-Bass.

Kelly, L., & Brown, J. B. (2002). Listening to native patients. Changes in physicians' understanding and behaviour. *Canadian Family Physician Medecin de Famille Canadien, 48*(10), 1645–1652.

Keysar, B., & Henly, A. S. (2002). Speakers' overestimation of their effectiveness. *Psychological Science, 13*(3), 207–212. http://dx.doi.org/10.1111/1467-9280.00439

King, G., Shaw, L., Orchard, C. A., & Miller, S. (2010). The interprofessional socialization and valuing scale: A tool for evaluating the shift toward collaborative care approaches in health care settings. *Work (Reading, Mass.), 35*(1), 77–85. http://dx.doi.org/10.3233/WOR-2010-0959

Klinzing, D., & Klinzing, D. (1985). *Communication for allied health professionals*. Dubuque, IA: Wm. C. Brown.

Knapp, M., & Hall, J. (2002). *Nonverbal communication in human interaction* (5th ed.). Toronto, ON: Thomson Learning.

Kruger, J., & Dunning, D. (1999). Unskilled and unaware of it: How difficulties in recognizing one's own incompetence lead to inflated self-assessments. *Journal of Personality and Social Psychology, 77*(6), 1121–1134. http://dx.doi.org/10.1037/0022-3514.77.6.1121

Leathard, A. (2003). Models for interprofessional collaboration. In A. Leathard (Ed.), *Interprofessional collaboration: From policy to practice in health and social care* (pp. 93–118). New York, NY: Routledge. http://dx.doi.org/10.4324/9780203420690_chapter_7

Lei, S. A., Rhinehart, P. J., Howard, H. A., & Cho, J. K. (2010). Strategies for improving reading comprehension among college students. *Reading Improvement, 47*, 30–42.

Leipzig, R. M., Hyer, K., Ek, K., et al. (2002). Attitudes toward working on interdisciplinary healthcare teams: A comparison by discipline. *Journal of the American Geriatrics Society, 50*(6), 1141–1148. http://dx.doi.org/10.1046/j.1532-5415.2002.50274.x

Levine, J. M., & Choi, H.-S. (2004). Impact of personnel turnover on team performance and cognition. In E. Salas & S. M. Fiore (Eds.), *Team cognition: Understanding the factors that drive process and performance* (pp. 153–176). Washington, DC: American Psychological Association. http://dx.doi.org/10.1037/10690-008

Levine, J. M., Choi, H., & Moreland, R. L. (2003). Newcomer innovation in work teams. In P. B. Paulus & B. A. Nijstad (Eds.), *Group creativity: Innovation through collaboration* (pp. 202–224). New York, NY: Oxford University Press. http://dx.doi.org/10.1093/acprof:oso/9780195147308.003.0010

Lev-On, A., Chavez, A., & Bicchieri, C. (2010). Group and dyadic communication in trust games. *Rationality and Society, 22*(1), 37–54. http://dx.doi.org/10.1177/1043463109337100

Lingard, L., Espin, S., Rubin, B., et al. (2005). Getting teams to talk: Development and pilot implementation of a checklist to promote interprofessional communication in the OR. *Quality & Safety in Health Care, 14*(5), 340–346. http://dx.doi.org/10.1136/qshc.2004.012377

Lingard, L., Regehr, G., Orser, B., et al. (2008). Evaluation of a preoperative checklist and team briefing among surgeons, nurses, and anesthesiologists to reduce failures in communication. *Archives of Surgery, 143*(1), 12–17. http://dx.doi.org/10.1001/archsurg.2007.21

Louie, B. Y., Drevdahl, D. J., Purdy, J. M., & Stackman, R. W. (2003). Advancing the scholarship of teaching through collaborative self-study. *Journal of Higher Education, 74*(2), 150–171. http://dx.doi.org/10.1353/jhe.2003.0016

Ludden, M. (2002). *Effective communication skills*. Indianapolis, IN: JIST Publishing.

Lukas, C. V., Mohr, D. C., & Meterko, M. (2009). Team effectiveness and organizational context in the implementation of a clinical innovation. *Quality Management in Health Care, 18*(1), 25–39. http://dx.doi.org/10.1097/01.QMH.0000344591.56133.90

Luor, T., Wu, L. L., Lu, H. P., & Tao, Y. H. (2010). The effect of emoticons in simplex and complex task-oriented communication: An empirical study of instant messaging. *Computers in Human Behavior, 26*, 889–895. http://dx.doi.org/10.1016/j.chb.2010.02.003

Lynch, B. (2006). Sharing information and confidentiality: Focused solutions in practice. *Community Practitioner, 79*(2), 53–55.

Mandy, A., Milton, C., & Mandy, P. (2004). Professional stereotyping and interprofessional education. *Learning in Health and Social Care, 3*(3), 154–170. http://dx.doi.org/10.1111/j.1473-6861.2004.00072.x

Margalef García, L., & Pareja Roblin, N. (2008). Innovation, research and professional development in higher education: Learning from our own experience. *Teaching and Teacher Education, 24*(1), 104–116. http://dx.doi.org/10.1016/j.tate.2007.03.007

Marshall, S., Harrison, J., & Flanagan, B. (2009). The teaching of a structured tool improves the clarity and content of interprofessional clinical communication. *Quality & Safety in Health Care, 18*(2), 137–140. http://dx.doi.org/10.1136/qshc.2007.025247

Mattessich, P. W., Murray-Close, M., & Monsey, B. R. (2001). *Collaboration: What makes it work?* (2nd ed.). St. Paul, MN: Fieldstone Alliance.

McClure, L. (2014). How to run a brainstorm for introverts (and extroverts too). TEDBlog. Retrieved from blog.ted.com/how-to-run-a-brainstorm-for-introverts-and-extroverts-too/

McCollom, M. (1990). Reevaluating group development: A critique of the familiar models. In J. Gillette & M. McCollom (Eds.), *Groups in context: A new perspective on group dynamics* (pp. 133–154). Reading, MA: Addison-Wesley.

McKay, M., Davis, M., & Fanning, P. (2009). *Messages: The communication skills book* (3rd ed.). Oakland, CA: New Harbinger.

McLeod, M. E. (2003). The caring physician: A journey in self-exploration and self-care. *American Journal of Gastroenterology, 98*(10), 2135–2138. http://dx.doi.org/10.1111/j.1572-0241.2003.07719.x

McNaughton, D., Hamlin, D., McCarthy, J., Head-Reeves, D., & Schreiner, M. (2008). Learning to listen: Teaching an active listening strategy to preservice education professionals. *Topics in Early Childhood Special Education, 27*(4), 223–231. http://dx.doi.org/10.1177/0271121407311241

McNaughton, D., & Vostal, B. R. (2010). Using active listening to improve collaboration with parents: The LAFF don't CRY strategy. *Intervention in School and Clinic, 45*(4), 251–256. http://dx.doi.org/10.1177/1053451209353443

Mill, J. S. (1848). *Principles of Political Economy with some of their Applications to Social Philosophy.* Book 3, Chapter 18, 7th edition published 1909, London, UK: Longmans, Green and Co. Retrieved from www.econlib.org/library/Mill/mlP46.html

Miller, J. N. (1965, September). The art of intelligent listening. *Reader's Digest, 127,* 83–86.

Mosser, G., & Begun, J. W. (2014). *Understanding teamwork in health care.* New York, NY: McGraw-Hill Education.

Motley, V., Reese, M. K., & Campos, P. (2014). Evaluating corrective feedback self-efficacy changes among counselor educators and site supervisors. *Counselor Education and Supervision, 53*(1), 34–46. http://dx.doi.org/10.1002/j.1556-6978.2014.00047.x

Napier, R. W., & Gershenfeld, M. K. (2004). *Groups: Theory and experience* (7th ed.). Boston, MA: Houghton Mifflin.

Nemerowicz, G., & Rosi, E. (1997). *Education for leadership and social responsibility.* London, UK: Falmer Press.

Orchard, C. A., King, G. A., Khalili, H., & Bezzina, M. B. (2012). Assessment of interprofessional team collaboration scale (AITCS): Development and testing of the instrument. *Journal of Continuing Education in the Health Professions, 32*(1), 58–67. http://dx.doi.org/10.1002/chp.21123

Paslawski, T. (2013). The perceptions of pre-service health science students of the barriers to interprofessional collaboration. *Journal of Educational Administration and Foundations, 23*(1), 65–71.

Patterson, K., Grenny, J., McMillan, R., & Switzler, A. (2012). *Crucial conversations.* New York, NY: McGraw-Hill.

Pearce, C. L., & Conger, J. A. (2003). All those years ago: The historical underpinnings of shared leadership. In C. L. Pearce & J. A. Conger (Eds.), *Shared leadership: Reframing the hows and whys of leadership* (pp. 1–18). Thousand Oaks, CA: Sage. http://dx.doi. org/10.4135/9781452229539.n1

Pentland, A. (2014). *Social Physics: How good ideas spread: The lessons from a new science.* New York, NY: Penguin.

Personal Strengths Publishing. (2015). *SDI & conflict.* Retrieved from www.strengthdeployment. com/sdi/sdi-and-conflict/

Porter, E. H. (1996). *Relationship awareness theory: Manual of administration and interpretation* (9th ed.). Carlsbad, CA: Personal Strengths Publishing.

Rashid, M., & Zimring, C. (2008). A review of the empirical literature on the relationships between indoor environment and stress in health care and office settings: Problems and prospects of sharing evidence. *Environment and Behavior, 40*(2), 151–190. http://dx.doi. org/10.1177/0013916507311550

Rees, C. E., & Garrud, P. (2001). Identifying undergraduate medical students' attitudes towards communication skills learning: A pilot study. *Medical Teacher, 23*(4), 400–406. http://dx.doi. org/10.1080/01421590120057067

Rees, C. E., Sheard, C. E., & McPherson, A. C. (2002). A qualitative study to explore undergraduate medical students' attitudes towards communication skills learning. *Medical Teacher, 24*(3), 289–293. http://dx.doi.org/10.1080/01421590220134123

Reeves, S., & Freeth, D. (2006). Re-examining the evaluation of interprofessional education for community mental health teams with a different lens: Understanding presage, process and product factors. *Journal of Psychiatric and Mental Health Nursing, 13*(6), 765–770. http:// dx.doi.org/10.1111/j.1365-2850.2006.01032.x

Rice, K., Zwarenstein, M., Conn, L. G., Kenaszchuk, C., Russell, A., & Reeves, S. (2010). An intervention to improve interprofessional collaboration and communications: A comparative qualitative study. *Journal of Interprofessional Care, 24*(4), 350–361. http://dx.doi. org/10.3109/13561820903550713

Rodgers, C. (2002). Defining reflection: Another look at John Dewey and reflective thinking. *Teachers College Record, 104*(4), 842–866. http://dx.doi.org/10.1111/1467-9620.00181

Roegiers, X. (2007). Curricular reforms guide schools: But, where to? *Prospects, 37*(2), 155–186. http://dx.doi.org/10.1007/s11125-007-9024-z

Rosen, M. A., Schiebel, N., Salas, E., Wu, T. S., Silvestri, S., & King, H. B. (2013). How can team performance be measured and diagnosed? In E. Salas & K. Frush (with D. P. Baker, J. B. Battles, H. B. King, & R. L. Wears) (Eds.), *Improving patient safety through teamwork and team training* (pp. 59–79). New York, NY: Oxford University.

Royal College of Physicians and Surgeons of Canada. (2005). *The CanMEDS 2005 Physician Competency Framework.* Retrieved from www.royalcollege.ca/portal/page/portal/rc/common/ documents/canmeds/resources/publications/framework_full_e.pdf

Salas, E., & Fiore, S. M. (2004). Why team cognition? An overview. In E. Salas & S. M. Fiore (Eds.), *Team cognition: Understanding the factors that drive process and performance* (pp. 3–8). Washington, DC: American Psychological Association. http://dx.doi.org/ 10.1037/10690-001

Salas, E., Wilson, K. A., Murphy, C. E., King, H., & Salisbury, M. (2008). Communicating, coordinating, and cooperating when lives depend on it: Tips for teamwork. *Joint Commission Journal on Quality and Patient Safety, 34*, 333–341.

Sarampalis, A., Kalluri, S., Edwards, B., & Hafter, E. (2009). Objective measures of listening effort: Effects of background noise and noise reduction. *Journal of Speech, Language, and Hearing Research: JSLHR, 52*(5), 1230–1240. http://dx.doi.org/10.1044/1092-4388(2009/08-0111)

Schmitt, M. H. (2001). Collaboration improves the quality of care: Methodological challenges and evidence from US health care research. *Journal of Interprofessional Care, 15*(1), 47–66. http:// dx.doi.org/10.1080/13561820020022873

Seaburn, D., Lorenz, A., Gunn, W., Gawinski, B., & Mauksch, L. (1996). *Models of collaboration: A guide for mental health professionals working with health care practitioners.* New York, NY: Basic Books.

Shokeir, V. (2008). Evidence for the stable use of uptalk in South Ontario English. *University of Pennsylvania Working Papers in Linguistics, 14*(2), 15–24. Retrieved from repository.upenn. edu/pwpl/vol14/iss2/4

Smith, M. K. (2005). *Bruce W. Tuckman: Forming, storming, norming and performing in groups.* The encyclopaedia of informal education. Retrieved from infed.org/mobi/bruce-w-tuckman-forming-storming-norming-and-performing-in-groups/

Sommers, L. S., Marton, K. I., Barbaccia, J. C., & Randolph, J. (2000). Physician, nurse, and social worker collaboration in primary care for chronically ill seniors. *Archives of Internal Medicine, 160*(12), 1825–1833. http://dx.doi.org/10.1001/archinte.160.12.1825

Spillane, J. P. (2005). Distributed leadership. *Educational Forum, 69*(2), 143–150. http://dx.doi. org/10.1080/00131720508984678

Stacey, D., Légaré, F., Col, N. F., Bennett, C. L., Barry, M. J., Eden, K. B., et al. (2014). Decision aids for people facing health treatment or screening decisions. Cochrane Database of Systematic Reviews Art. No.: CD001431. doi:10.1002/14651858.CD001431.pub4.

Stewart, M. (2001). Towards a global definition of patient centred care. *BMJ (Clinical Research Ed.), 322*(7284), 444–445. Retrieved from www.ncbi.nlm.nih.gov/pmc/articles/PMC1119673/. http://dx.doi.org/10.1136/bmj.322.7284.444

Straus, D. (2002). *How to make collaboration work: Powerful ways to build consensus, solve problems, and make decisions.* San Francisco, CA: Berrett-Koehler.

Suter, E., Deutschlander, S., & Lait, J. (2011). Using a complex systems perspective to achieve sustainable health care practice change. *Journal of Research in Interprofessional Practice and Education, 2*(1), 83–99.

Thomas, K. W. (1976). Conflict and conflict management. In M. D. Dunnette (Ed.), *Handbook of industrial and organizational psychology* (pp. 889–935). Chicago, IL: Rand McNally.

Thomas, K. W. (1992). Conflict and conflict management: Reflections and update. *Journal of Organizational Behavior, 13*(3), 265–274. http://dx.doi.org/10.1002/job.4030130307

Thomas, K.W., Fann Thomas, G., & Schaubhut, N. (2008). Conflict styles of men and women at six organization levels. *International Journal of Conflict Management, 19*(2), 148–166. http://dx.doi.org/10.1108/10444060810856085

Thomas, K. W., & Kilmann, R. H. (2007). Thomas-Kilman conflict mode instrument: Profile and interpretative report. Retrieved from www.kilmanndiagnostics.com/sites/default/files/TKI_Sample_Report.pdf

Tuckman, B. W. (1965). Developmental sequence in small groups. *Psychological Bulletin, 63*(6), 384–399. http://dx.doi.org/10.1037/h0022100

Ünal, S. (2012). Evaluating the effect of self-awareness and communication techniques on nurses' assertiveness and self-esteem. *Contemporary Nurse, 43*(1), 90–98. http://dx.doi.org/10.5172/conu.2012.43.1.90

Vroom, V. H. (2000). Leadership and the decision-making process. *Organizational Dynamics, 28*(4), 82–94. http://dx.doi.org/10.1016/S0090-2616(00)00003-6

Waber, B. N., Olguin Olguin, D., Kim, T., & Pentland, A. (2010). Productivity through coffee breaks: Changing social networks by changing break structure. http://dx.doi.org/10.2139/ssrn.1586375

Wagner, E. H., & Groves, T. (2002). Care for chronic diseases: The efficacy of coordinated and patient centred care is established, but now is the time to test its effectiveness. *BMJ: British Medical Journal, 325*(7370), 913. Retrieved from www.ncbi.nlm.nih.gov/pmc/articles/PMC1124427/

Warshawsky, N. E., Havens, D. S., & Knafl, G. (2012). The influence of interpersonal relationships on nurse managers' work engagement and proactive work behavior. *Journal of Nursing Administration, 42*(9), 418–425. http://dx.doi.org/10.1097/NNA.0b013e3182668129

Way, D. O., Jones, L., & Busing, N. (2000). *Implementation strategies: Collaboration in primary care: Family doctors & nurse practitioners delivering shared care.* Discussion paper written for the Ontario College of Family Physicians. Retrieved from http://www.eicp.ca/en/toolkit/hhr/ocfp-paper-handout.pdf

Weger, H., Jr., Castle, G. R., & Emmett, M. C. (2010). Active listening in peer interviews: The influence of message paraphrasing on perceptions of listening skill. *International Journal of Listening, 24*(1), 34–49. http://dx.doi.org/10.1080/10904010903466311

Wertheimer, J. C., Roebuck-Spencer, T. M., Constantinidou, F., Turkstra, L., Pavol, M., & Paul, D. (2008). Collaboration between neuropsychologists and speech-language pathologists in rehabilitation settings. *Journal of Head Trauma Rehabilitation, 23*(5), 273–285. http://dx.doi.org/10.1097/01.HTR.0000336840.76209.a1

Whitehead, C. (2007). The doctor dilemma in interprofessional education and care: How and why will physicians collaborate? *Medical Education, 41*(10), 1010–1016. http://dx.doi.org/10.1111/j.1365-2923.2007.02893.x

World Health Organization. (2007). Look-alike, sound-alike medication names. *Patient Safety Solutions, 1*(1). Retrieved from www.who.int/patientsafety/solutions/patientsafety/PS-Solution1.pdf

World Health Organization. (2009). *Surgical Safety Checklist.* Retrieved from www.who.int/patientsafety/safesurgery/checklist/en/

World Health Organization. (2010). *Framework for action on interprofessional education and collaborative practice.* Retrieved from http://www.who.int/hrh/resources/framework_action/en/

Wynia, M. K., Von Kohorn, I., & Mitchell, P. H. (2012). Challenges at the intersection of team-based and patient-centered health care: Insights from an IOM working group. *Journal of the American Medical Association, 308*(13), 1327–1328. http://dx.doi.org/10.1001/jama.2012.12601

Yeatts, D. E., & Hyten, C. (1998). *High-performing self-managed work teams: A comparison of theory to practice.* Thousand Oaks, CA: Sage. http://dx.doi.org/10.4135/9781483328218

Youker, R. (2013). Using the communications styles instrument for teambuilding. *PM World Journal, 2*(7) 1–18. Retrieved from pmworldlibrary.net/wp-content/uploads/2013/07/pmwj12-jul2013-youker-communication-styles-SecondEdition.pdf

Zorek, J., & Raehl, C. (2013). Interprofessional education accreditation standards in the USA: A comparative analysis. *Journal of Interprofessional Care, 27*(2), 123–130. http://dx.doi.org/10.3109/13561820.2012.718295

Zwarenstein, M., Goldman, J., & Reeves, S. (2009). Interprofessional collaboration: Effects of practice-based interventions on professional practice and healthcare outcomes. *Cochrane Database of Systematic Reviews* Art. No. CD000072. doi:10.1002/14651858.CD000072.pub2.

Zwarenstein, M., Reeves, S., & Perrier, L. (2005). Effectiveness of pre-licensure interprofessional education and post-licensure collaborative interventions. *Journal of Interprofessional Care, 19*(s1 S1), 148–165. http://dx.doi.org/10.1080/13561820500082800

Zwarenstein, M., Reeves, S., Russell, A., et al. (2007). Structuring communication relationships for interprofessional teamwork (SCRIPT): A cluster randomized controlled trial. *Trials, 8*(23). Retrieved from www.trialsjournal.com/content/8/1/23

Zwarenstein, M., Rice, K., Gotlib-Conn, L., Kenaszchuk, C., & Reeves, S. (2013). Disengaged: A qualitative study of communication and collaboration between physicians and other professions on general internal medicine wards. *BMC Health Services Research, 13*(1), 494. Retrieved from www.biomedcentral.com/1472-6963/13/494. http://dx.doi.org/10.1186/1472-6963-13-494

Index

About the Authors

Deborah Lake is a clinical psychologist with a BA with Distinction in Psychology from the University of Delaware and an MA and PhD in Psychology from the University of Waterloo. Over the past 40 years, Deborah has collaborated with other professionals in school systems in North Carolina and Ontario and in mental health services, pediatric outpatient clinics, and public health services in Saskatchewan. She has led workshops on interprofessional collaboration for educators and health professionals, including clinical teams of the National Centre for Operational Stress Injuries, Veterans Affairs Canada. Deborah taught and supervised psychology students and other healthcare trainees as a Professional Affiliate with the College of Graduate Studies and Research at the University of Saskatchewan from 1986 to 2011, and she is currently an Assistant Professor in the Clinical Health Psychology Department at the University of Manitoba.

Krista Baerg is a consultant pediatrician and associate professor of pediatrics at the University of Saskatchewan. Her clinical interests include interdisciplinary practice, patient- and family-centered care, pain management, and quality improvement. She completed her BScMed and MD as well as her specialty training in pediatrics at the University of Saskatchewan. She has worked with interdisciplinary teams in both acute care and outpatient settings at a teaching hospital. Prior to entering medicine, she completed a BSN and worked as a nurse in remote northern communities.

Teresa Paslawski is a faculty member in Communication Sciences and Disorders, Faculty of Rehabilitation Medicine at the University of Alberta. One of her main research interests is the scholarship of teaching and learning. In addition to teaching and doing research in speech language pathology, she is actively involved in interprofessional education training and contributes to the Master of Education in Health Sciences Education Program at the University of Alberta. Teresa has a BA *(Summa Cum Laude)* in Speech-Language Pathology from Minot State

University, North Dakota, an MA in Speech Language Pathology from the University of California, Santa Barbara, and a PhD in Neuroscience (Psychiatry) from the University of Alberta. She has done postdoctoral fellowships in Neurology at the University of Alberta Hospital in Edmonton and in Speech Pathology at the Mayo Clinic in Rochester, Minnesota. She has worked clinically in acute care, acute and outpatient rehabilitation primarily with adults with neurological disorders.